THE HAY DIET
MADE EASY

THE HAY DIET MADE EASY

A Practical Guide to Food Combining
with advice on
medically unrecognised illness

JACKIE HABGOOD
Drawings by Alexandra Habgood

SOUVENIR PRESS

First published 1997 by Souvenir Press Ltd, 43 Great Russell Street, London WC1B 3PA

Reprinted 1997 (three times)
Reprinted 1998 (four times)

ISBN 0 285 63379 1

Photoset by Rowland Phototypesetting Ltd, Bury St Edmunds, Suffolk.
Printed in Great Britain by
The Guernsey Press Company Ltd,
Guernsey, Channel Islands.

To anyone who would like a simpler guide to the Hay diet

To those who wish to improve their general health

To anyone who finds it impossible to keep to a diet
however hard they try

To people wishing to maximise their potential,
mentally, physically and intellectually

And to the many people suffering with a long list of
unexplained symptoms

I dedicate this book

ABOUT THE AUTHOR

Jackie Habgood worked until her first daughter was born in 1976, when her health began to deteriorate. Over the next ten years she became increasingly tired and exhausted and accumulated an endless list of mental and physical symptoms. All the tests and examinations were negative, nothing her doctor knew, and nothing she herself had learnt as a health visitor, seemed to help. After six years she was given antidepressant drugs.

Then, from her own reading, she discovered the answers: they were straightforward and they lay in her diet. Her illness could have been avoided by very simple measures and attention to her diet could have prevented the need for drugs. She has gradually recovered her strength using the methods described in this book.

Acknowledgements

My grateful thanks to the growing number of doctors and dietitians who are opening their minds to this approach.

The case histories described in the book are all true accounts of individual experiences, but for the sake of confidentiality names have been altered. A big thank-you to all those who have generously given their permission for their stories to be included.

Above all, this book has been a family effort. My love and thanks go to Ken for his practical support, to Alexandra for the drawings and to Chloe for her help with the word processor.

J.H.

Contents

Note to Readers

Every care has been taken to ensure that the instructions and advice given in this book are accurate and practical. However, where health is concerned—and in particular a serious problem of any kind—I must stress that there is no substitute for seeking advice from a qualified medical practitioner. All persistent symptoms, of whatever nature, may have underlying causes that need, and should not be treated without, professional elucidation and evaluation. It is therefore very important, if you intend to use this book for self-help, only to do so in conjunction with duly prescribed conventional or other therapy. In any event, read the advice carefully, and pay particular attention to the precautions and warnings.

The Publisher makes no representation, express or implied, with regard to the accuracy of the information contained in this book, and legal responsibility or liability cannot be accepted by the Author or the Publisher for any errors or omissions that may be made or for any loss, damage, injury or problems suffered or in any way arising from following the nutritional advice offered in these pages.

Jackie Habgood
February 1997

Preface

This book is intended as a practical guide for busy people. I have developed it through teaching the Hay diet and through counselling, and it has proved to be the most exciting and rewarding project I have ever undertaken, especially since I find that about one in every ten Hay-dieters achieves quite spectacular results. The content of the book is built on what I have learned from their hard work and experience.

If you have ever attempted to follow the Hay diet, you will know that it consists of a few basic ideas which can sometimes be quite difficult to put into practice. Food combining does require a lot of understanding and a lot of commitment, however easy anyone tries to make it, but I have tried to help you solve any problems you may encounter and the results will give you all the encouragement you need. Everything is simplified and all the meals are worked out, right down to the sandwiches and the lunchboxes. Just choose from the lists of meals and snacks or select from the menus at the end of the book.

But this is not just another Hay diet book. It is a powerful healing programme, designed to open your eyes to the many things you can do to assist in your own recovery.

When I started teaching the Hay diet I found that almost everyone on my courses was suffering to some extent from medically unrecognised illness. Nine out of ten were affected by low blood sugar, and at least twenty per cent were also suffering from candida, yet most of them had no idea why they felt unwell.

LOW BLOOD SUGAR (HYPOGLYCAEMIA)
This is a controversial and very much misunderstood problem. Hardly anyone realises how widespread it is or what it can lead to if it is neglected, and very few people indeed know how simply it

can be relieved. It may surprise you to learn that sugar is not the answer.

CANDIDA

This common and very debilitating yeast or thrush infection is caused by the great changes in our diet and lifestyle during the twentieth century. The list of mental and physical symptoms may be endless. Tests and examinations often prove negative and no one seems able to help, yet candida too is a treatable condition.

UNSUSPECTED FOOD INTOLERANCES

Food intolerance is another major cause of unexplained fatigue and chronic illness of every kind—everyday foods are responsible for more trouble than anyone realises. This problem too is extremely widespread but seldom recognised. The Hay diet will usually expose any major troublemakers, and problems which have persisted for many years can often be substantially relieved in a comparatively short time.

So if you are not as well as you would like, this book will help you to take the first essential step on the road to recovery by changing your diet. It is an exciting and positive approach, and psychologically it works wonders.

J.H.

CHAPTER 1

Introducing the Hay Diet

The Hay diet takes its name from Dr William Howard Hay (1866–1940), an American surgeon who had to give up practising at the age of forty when he suffered a complete breakdown in health. At sixteen stone he was so ill with heart trouble, high blood pressure and serious kidney disease that he was not expected to live. In desperation he turned to the teachings of the early American naturopaths.

As every naturopath knows, if we give our own body the right conditions it will come to our aid, releasing its own remarkable healing power. All we have to do is give it the raw material to do the job and take away everything that hinders its work. This means a completely natural diet, with plenty of fresh fruit and vegetables; at the same time processed foods like sugar and white flour have to go because they block the healing process. The body is then free to devote all its energy to the fight against illness.

Dr Hay therefore ate 'fundamentally', that is, he restricted himself to fresh fruit and vegetables, whole grains, fresh meat and fish—and he confounded his doctors by recovering in three months. By this time he had lost three stone in weight and after twelve months he was back to an active life.

Over the next 26 years Dr Hay treated all his patients naturally. They came to him from right across the world and many of those who recovered had been thought to be incurable. He led a very busy life, without an ache or a pain, until the age of seventy-four when he died tragically after a serious accident.

Our diet has changed dramatically for the worse since the 1930s when Dr Hay wrote his best-selling book, *A New Health Era*. Food was more natural then, so it was very much easier to adapt to his diet, but with a little effort it is still possible to follow it today.

WHAT ARE THE RULES?

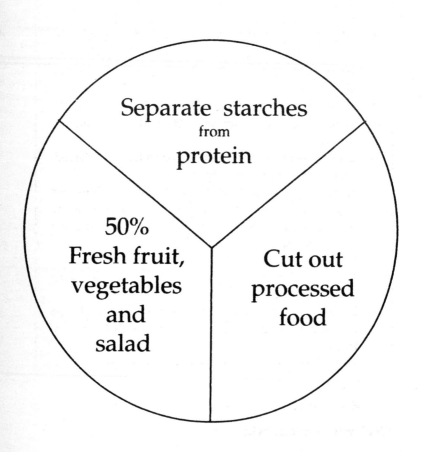

Separate starches from protein

50% Fresh fruit, vegetables and salad

Cut out processed food

WHAT CAN THE HAY DIET DO FOR ME?

- It relieves stress.
- It can add hours to your day.
- It improves efficiency and heightens mental performance.
- It clears your skin and conditions your hair.
- It restores your weight to normal and keeps it that way.
- It strengthens natural immunity: colds and viruses are usually short-lived and can often be avoided altogether.
- Sports enthusiasts and people whose work is physically demanding find it improves their stamina and endurance.
- Chronic pain can sometimes be considerably relieved, especially the pain of arthritis.
- It enhances medical treatment and other therapies such as homoeopathy. If you use it before an operation you will be surprised at how much you can help yourself while you wait.
- It speeds recovery from illness, operation or injury.
- It offers a longer and more active life, and reduces the fear of serious disease.
- If you have had cancer, this diet of safe, natural food can do much to restore your strength and peace of mind.

THE HAY DIET

'Don't mix foods that fight'

Food combining is an idea that Dr Hay adopted after his recovery and he used it with great success. Starchy foods like bread and potatoes are never eaten with concentrated protein foods like meat and cheese: they are taken at separate meals because they have opposite digestive requirements. This is the first step in the Hay diet and it can bring surprising improvements, often in a very short time.

The Hay diet is a high-energy diet, providing the extra vitality and drive needed to cope with a very busy life. It is the high raw-food diet often used on continental health farms to cleanse and revive people at great expense. It is definitely the diet of the future.

Grow old gracefully—why not?

At a Hay diet banquet not long ago I met several elderly Hay-dieters who were striking proof of the power of this diet. They were fit, they were alert, and most of them proved to be ten or fifteen years older than I would ever have guessed. Doris Grant, co-author of *Food Combining for Health*, has been following the Hay diet herself for the past sixty years, and she brought out another book in her ninety-first year.

WHY SUFFER?

There is absolutely no need to be a helpless victim of any illness. If you are one of the many people whose health has mysteriously deteriorated over the years, yet no one can identify your problem, why not investigate your diet? The Hay diet will often relieve long-standing problems in cases where nothing else has ever really helped. Whatever your situation, you can still obtain substantial improvements.

ALL THESE RESPOND VERY WELL

Indigestion	Eczema
Peptic ulcers	Asthma
Irritable bowel	Arthritis
Colitis	Migraine
Chronic fatigue	Candida
M.E. (myalgic encephalomyelitis)	

If your problem is not mentioned in this list, remember that the Hay diet begins to restore normal function whatever the cause of the trouble because it triggers our own natural healing mechanism. With our support and understanding the body soon gets on with the job of healing and repair, using its own marvellous intelligence. This is strong medicine: the effect is lasting and the improvement is continuous.

THE HAY DIET IS CONTROVERSIAL

Our knowledge of nutrition is still elementary and many aspects remain unexplained, but there is plenty of living proof that the Hay diet works, and that's what really counts. Scientific proof is by no means essential for a safe and simple remedy like this, but do not be surprised if your doctor fails to take it seriously—it does not always make much sense to a scientific mind! Dietitians have a scientific training too, so most of them react in a similar way. However the opinions of those who have adopted the diet speak for themselves.

The voices of experience

No more processed food for me. I feel so much fresher, lighter, I'd never go back to the old way of eating. I love all the vegetables and I never miss my potato at lunchtime.

I've felt better right from the start. I'm much more alert and I wake much earlier now. My husband said, 'You'll never get anywhere on this diet, you're always eating', but I've lost five pounds in the last three weeks without really trying.

I've never felt better in myself. I feel just like I did when I was eighteen, and now I can drive my lorry without having to stop for snacks. The unloading is the heavy part, but I manage it very much better on this diet.

This is not just another diet, my heartburn improved straight away and my arthritic knees are much less painful.

ECZEMA AND ASTHMA

'You're not STILL on that diet, are you?'

'It's not really a diet, it's the way I live now.'

In three months Sandra has lost a stone in weight. She has stopped wheezing and thrown her inhaler away, and the eczema has gradually gone. And that's not all: she's so much happier and more alert these days; she's delighted, and who wouldn't be?

GOODBYE TO ACNE

Jonathan had been living on a student diet of junk food for a very long time and his face was a mass of septic spots. He worked really hard on the Hay diet and, to his great surprise, all the spots healed in just four weeks. The smooth red patches which remained have gradually disappeared without trace.

NO MORE PAIN

George had had a duodenal ulcer for thirty years and for the last fourteen of them had been taking a very expensive remedy for the pain. He was a real sugarholic: he ate sweets and chocolate biscuits all day long and would even wake up for a snack in the night. But since he has been eating two-hourly on the Hay diet the pain has improved a lot and the bloating has gone down. He was slimmer round the middle after only a week. His wife Anne comments:

'He hasn't had a twinge of stomach pain for the last five weeks, and that's a record. He had pain every day and it was awful, terrible, yet he has not needed a single ulcer tablet and now he sleeps right through for at least six hours every night, something which has not happened in sixteen years. He's lost fourteen pounds in four weeks without even feeling hungry and he's got lots more energy too.'

George has since found that root vegetables bring the pain back. Ulcer pain is often related to particular foods.

LIFE AFTER CANCER

At the age of seventy-seven Amelia was struggling to recover from an operation for bowel cancer six months before. She was frightened, and every little pain put her in a panic. She could hardly walk the fifty yards to the shops and felt that this must be the end of her life. Then, as she watched a friend's despair over arthritis turning to hope on the Hay diet, she wanted to know more. She studied Dr Hay's original book, *A New Health Era*, and was hooked.

She adapted her life very quickly and after three weeks' hard work was able to do three hours' gardening. She recovered from the first of the winter infections in just a day and now looks and feels a thousand times better. She is no longer afraid and is looking forward to many more years of active life. 'I've totally changed my lifestyle; I felt better right from the start and I'm finding it all a great adventure.'

Food Combining for Life by Doris Grant contains many more remarkable success stories and you may discover how someone else has recovered from your own particular problem.

HERE'S HEALTH
Have you experienced it?

A trim figure

Clear skin

Shining hair

Sound sleep, early waking

Strength and stamina

A comfortable body

A clear head

Good concentration

A good memory

An optimistic outlook

Emotional stability

A ready smile

If you are in this happy situation, you can use the Hay diet to maintain it for the rest of your life. If you are wilting, you will be surprised at how quickly you start to blossom again. And if you have forgotten what it is like to feel well, be patient and work hard on your diet; you can improve your lot enormously. Dr Hay understood that we cannot recover completely until we learn to rebuild our own health.

CHAPTER 2

Beat Low Blood Sugar

Most of us know when our blood sugar is low. It's a familiar feeling: our concentration slips, we get tired and irritable, and we need something to pick us up. If we are well and if our body chemistry is well balanced, it only happens if a meal is late or if we miss a meal, but on today's diet of highly processed food it can happen more and more often until we come to depend on a regular supply of tea or coffee and biscuits to help us through the day. Few people realise that the sugar and stimulants which pick us up are also responsible for the tiredness that follows later.

Hypoglycaemia or low blood sugar was first identified by an American GP, Dr Seale Harris, in 1924, shortly after insulin was introduced. He very soon realised that not only his diabetic patients were suffering from 'hypo' attacks; many other people, who were not diabetics at all, were also experiencing them. But to this day the treatment of everyday hypoglycaemia is still not part of a doctor's training. Like everyone else, many GPs still believe that sugar is the remedy, and in my experience few health practitioners recognise the huge extent of the problem either.

Some of us find that the Hay diet solves the problem entirely. It stabilises blood sugar levels automatically because it consists of natural foods which are themselves whole and perfectly balanced. Our energy comes back, and we are delighted.

Others find they need more help:
    'Dieting makes me feel sinking and ill.'
    'Diets don't work for me. I've tried them all but I never lose weight.'
        'I can't possibly give up sugar, I binge . . . I'm a chocoholic.'
        'I get tired and depressed, I eat for comfort.'

Diets can be difficult or impossible to keep to unless you have a good understanding of blood sugar, and few of us have.

But surely we need sugar for energy—it's natural, isn't it?
This is what advertisers lead us to believe, but we know little of its true effects. People who are always tired may take more sugar and stimulants than anyone else in an effort to keep going, but actually they make the problem worse.

These are the biggest offenders:
- Sugar.
- All sweetened foods: biscuits, ice-cream, cakes, chocolate, sweet desserts.
- White bread and white flour.
- Caffeine: coffee, tea. Soft drinks, especially cola.
- Concentrated natural fruit juice—dilute it.
- Tobacco and alcohol.

All these, taken to excess, can so exhaust the liver, pancreas and adrenal glands that we are no longer able to keep our blood sugar levels steady. Sugar and stimulants have to be cut right out to give the system a chance to rest and recover. You will be very surprised at the relief this can bring.

But be careful!

If you are drinking a lot of tea, coffee or cola, or if your diet is high in sugar and sweetened foods, cut them down slowly enough to minimise the withdrawal symptoms. Headaches, stomach aches, tiredness and light-headedness are not uncommon. And whenever you cut anything out of the diet, always replace it with something natural which you enjoy.

Some people become very dependent on sugar. If you are already very debilitated and you change your diet too quickly, it may leave you feeling very weak and unwell, but this soon passes if you eat two-hourly, remembering to include plenty of natural starch foods, especially whole grains.

HOW LONG CAN YOU GO WITHOUT FOOD?

Low blood sugar is so common these days that few Hay-dieters can happily wait four hours between meals.

Snack on something neutral:
- Avocado pear, avocado cream.
- A few nuts or seeds with a raw carrot or celery stick.
- Salad of any kind.

Other snacks
- A glass of milk.
- If hunger strikes near to a protein-based meal, snack on acid fruit.
- Shortly before or after a starch meal you could have one of the sweeter fruits. Make sure it is firm and not too ripe.

SUGAR BLUES?

Is this you or your child?
Tense, nervous, insecure?
Aimless, apathetic, bored?

ARE YOU . . .
Forgetful and indecisive?
Tired and lacking in energy?
Moody, unhappy, mysteriously stressed?
Emotional and easily hurt?
Is it difficult to concentrate?

A treadmill existence
Is life hard, dull and boring?
Is it all work and no play?

These are early-warning symptoms of hypoglycaemia

A surprising number of us suffer from 'sugar blues': low blood sugar levels sap our energies and numb our spirit. When blood sugar levels are always low, when we are always 'hypo', we lose our drive and our ambition, we become bored, disorganised and dissatisfied with life, we lose our direction and fall into a rut. We slow down and the practical side of life becomes a problem—everything seems too much trouble. We find it difficult to get things done and resent having to do the chores. Low blood sugar takes away our confidence and destroys our self-esteem.

This state of affairs is so common nowadays that we stoically accept it as part of our lot. There may be no spectacular symptoms but it can still have a devastating effect on our lives. Yet changing the diet at this stage can be highly successful: people often find that their energy and optimism come flooding back in a very short time, sometimes in a matter of days.

THIS IS A 'HYPO' ATTACK

That sinking feeling!
Your blood sugar level is dropping fast
Sudden intense hunger
A swimming head
Difficulty focusing, blurred vision
Sudden tiredness

More severe attacks
Nausea
Sweating, shaking, panic
A racing heart

These attacks can leave you
tired and washed out for hours
YOU CAN LEARN TO AVOID THEM

Sugar is definitely not the answer, neither is glucose

They do pick us up of course, but they very soon let us down, leaving us gasping for another 'fix'. We are not naturally designed to deal with sugar once it has been taken out of the plant: it is too rich, too concentrated; it is like running a car with the choke out. It rapidly floods the system, short-circuiting normal body functions and sending blood sugar levels soaring. This is what gives us the initial lift.

The pancreas is then forced to produce an excessive amount of insulin to lower blood sugar as fast as possible, a panic measure to avoid the danger of coma. If you suffer from hypo attacks you can feel it happening. Blackouts and fainting are not uncommon in this situation.

By contrast, natural wholefoods release their sugar slowly and evenly into the bloodstream, keeping us on an even keel mentally and physically. They are our natural fuel; they are the only foods we can handle efficiently.

- Glucose is more refined than sugar, so it is even more rapidly absorbed.
- Stimulants like caffeine, tobacco and alcohol have similarly disruptive effects.

BUT I NEVER TAKE SUGAR!
All the hidden sugar in cakes, biscuits, chocolate, ice-cream and especially soft drinks is the main cause of the trouble, of course.

ARE YOU ON A RESTRICTED DIET?
People sometimes experience symptoms of hypoglycaemia and 'hypo' attacks for the first time when they begin a restricted diet for food allergy or candida (see Chapter 3), despite never taking any sugar or sweet foods, or stimulants of any kind. Usually they have no idea what these feelings are or what causes them. The most common reason is that they have cut down too much on concentrated starch foods like whole grains, not realising how much complex carbohydrate food they need if they are to keep their blood sugar level steady.

CHRONIC HYPOGLYCAEMIA

This has become a serious and incapacitating problem for many people. Those who have long suspected that their blood sugar is low may be baffled when blood sugar tests done at their doctor's surgery prove negative, misleading doctor and patient into believing that after all the problem lies somewhere else. But single tests are not actually very significant where low blood sugar is concerned; it takes a six-hour glucose tolerance test to diagnose hypoglycaemia and this is only available privately on a very limited basis. However, the effect of removing sugar and stimulants from the diet is usually so swift and so convincing that expensive testing is unnecessary.

Not all in the mind

Chronic hypoglycaemia is a major cause of mental and physical illness, so don't let yourself be labelled neurotic. People who have some knowledge of low blood sugar may nevertheless still not recognise that this could be their own problem. I did not myself. People with M.E. (myalgic encephalomyelitis) and chronic fatigue in particular may be quite severely affected. The books about low blood sugar which are recommended at the end of this book may come as a revelation. You could be very surprised indeed by what you read.

The root of the problem

When blood sugar is low, the oxygen supply to body, brain and nervous system is reduced. Glucose and oxygen burn together in body cells to produce energy, so where there is a lack of glucose, there is also a lack of oxygen. This is why such a wide variety of symptoms can result (see boxed list, p. 24).

THESE ARE SYMPTOMS OF CHRONIC HYPOGLYCAEMIA

Constant hunger	Constant tiredness
Headaches	Tension, PMT
Irritability	Poor concentration
Mood swings	Forgetfulness
Palpitations	A swimming head
Sleeping problems	Mental tiredness
Hot or cold sweats	Depression
Night sweats	Anxiety, panics
Aggression	Nightmares
Cold hands and feet	Apprehension
Cramps of all kinds	Drowsiness
Muscle weakness	Fainting, blackouts
Chronic indigestion	Constant worrying
Menstrual cramps	Mental confusion
Loss of appetite	Eating problems
Low sex drive	Stubborn weight problems

Routine medical tests usually prove negative

A treatable condition

Once they have removed sugar and stimulants from the diet and are eating naturally, many people recover from quite severe symptoms, especially if they are young and their diet has been very poor.

- Keep to the principles of the Hay diet.
- Be sure to snack between meals.
- Keep the concentrated starches and proteins separated. You may have to bring the starch meals and the protein meals closer together.

The blood sugar level drops overnight
- A carbohydrate snack before bedtime will help to keep it up so that you relax better and sleep longer.
- If you wake in the night, another starchy snack could send you straight back to sleep. You should wake feeling stronger and more ready to get up.
- A good starch-based breakfast can revive you if you wake up tired, and will sustain you through the morning. Porridge is a good idea.

This is the modern treatment for chronic hypoglycaemia

A diet high in complex carbohydrates brings swift and lasting relief and helps to correct the imbalance permanently. This has been my own experience and that of many others.

Complex carbohydrates form an integral part of natural whole foods:
- Jacket potatoes, fresh vegetables.
- Whole grains, including:
    natural brown rice, porridge oats, millet.
    wholemeal bread, wholemeal pasta.
- Peas, beans and lentils (in moderation).

A high natural carbohydrate/low animal protein diet
This is the diet recommended by Dr Paavo Airola in *Hypoglycaemia: A Better Approach*. It is easy to adapt it for vegetarians.

MORE SUSTAINING COMBINATIONS OF FOOD

The combinations of vegetarian foods which go together to make a complete protein are also a great help in stabilising blood sugar levels.
They are given in the table on page 92.

WHAT ABOUT HIGH-PROTEIN DIETS?
High-protein diets which are low in starch were originally used to treat hypoglycaemia, but although they do control the symptoms they are nutritionally unsound and it has since been found that they lead to more problems, including degenerative disease in the long term.

AVOID THE SWEETEST FRUITS
Bananas, dried fruits, sweet pears and sweet grapes may also cause blood sugar swings if you are very sensitive. The firmer, less ripe fruits may not affect you if they are taken in moderation.

Smaller meals, more often

Certain people who have suffered for a long time may obtain substantial relief by removing sugar and stimulants from their diet but nevertheless still suffer hypo attacks and remain unwell. Digesting average-size meals can be exhausting if you are very debilitated, and you may find that you function better on much smaller meals—mini-meals—taken approximately every two to three hours. This is the way I live myself: I concentrate better and I get much more work done this way. Here are some suggestions to get you started:

MINI-MEALS

STARCH-BASED MEALS	PROTEIN-BASED MEALS
Porridge	Egg salad
Wholemeal crispbreads	Natural yoghurt
Wholemeal roll or sandwich	Sliced meat and salad
Jacket potato	Celery and cheese
Hearty vegetable soup	Chicken leg and salad
Corn on the cob	Fish with salad

Eat every two to three hours
Spread the food out evenly over the day
Eat plenty of salad with or in between these meals
There are more ideas in Chapter 12

People with severe chronic hypoglycaemia are like a battery which cannot hold a charge; they have to eat little and often. As Dr Hay pointed out, the body has a great need for economy: keep this in mind, it will help you a lot. Listen to your body very carefully on this because even a little more food than you need can tire you out. You will be very surprised at how much more energy you can release by eating this way.

- Time the snacks to avoid the hypo attacks. It may be some time before you recover enough to avoid the tiredness that follows later.
- You will need two starch-based meals to every protein meal. Protein cannot be used efficiently in the body without sufficient starch.
- Starch and protein snacks are acid-forming so don't forget to maintain your alkaline balance with plenty of salad. Avocado cream is a refreshing treat.
- Remember to drink between meals. There is a list of natural drinks on p. 110.
- You should not put on weight by eating this way, in fact frequent snacking can be a good way to slim.
- If you are already slender, watch your weight and make sure you get enough to eat.

As you recover you will be able to wait a little longer between meals.

The road to recovery

Many other factors play a part in severe chronic hypoglycaemia, including:

- Unsuspected food intolerances.
- Hormone imbalance.
- Vitamin and mineral deficiencies.
- A deficiency of essential fatty acids.
- Rarely: more serious disease including tumours of the pancreas.

It is tempting to treat yourself, but if you are very unwell it is safer to get professional help if you possibly can, from a nutritional therapist, a naturopath, or from a doctor who specialises in nutritional medicine, so that you can deal with the underlying causes. Everybody's problem is different and with expert help you could make a faster recovery.

This chapter is just a quick guide. It is a simplified introduction to a complex and controversial subject, meant to open your eyes to the effects of low blood sugar. It is intended merely to help you identify the problem and to take the first essential steps to relieve it by changing your diet.

CHAPTER 3

Is Candida Your Problem?

Although candida as described in this chapter has been recognised since about 1983 by health practitioners and by doctors who specialise in nutritional medicine, this condition, like low blood sugar, is still not officially accepted as a problem by the medical profession in general. It is in any case a natural inhabitant of the body and there is as yet no completely reliable test for it; the diagnosis has to be based on your medical history and symptoms and on your response to treatment.

Harmless candida yeast lives on the skin and in everybody's gut, and before the development of the food industry, when food was more natural, it never caused much trouble; but when it is fed too much sugar or alcohol it can multiply out of control, and if it is neglected it may turn into an aggressive fungal infection. These fungi put down roots which pierce the lining of the gut so that candida toxins escape into the bloodstream and affect the whole system, causing a great variety of mental and physical symptoms.

A stressful life further lowers resistance to it, and a major stressful event may prove to be the last straw. Candida has become a huge problem because it is usually untreated; some people have suffered for many years, even a lifetime, and children too may be victims. If you suffer from several of the symptoms listed in the box on page 30, you may well have candida.

Other symptoms include:
- Cravings for sugar, bread, yeast or alcohol.
- Bubbling sensations in the intestines.
- Fungal infections of the skin or nails, athlete's foot.
- Reactions to perfume or tobacco smoke.
- Symptoms which become worse in damp or mouldy places.

THIS IS CHRONIC CANDIDA

Catarrh	Headaches
Furred mouth	Depression
Thrush in the mouth	Rashes, urticaria, itching
Persistent sore throat	Itchy anus, vulva, vagina
Indigestion, heartburn	Persistent vaginal thrush
Bloating, belching	Hot flushes
Embarrassing, offensive wind	Fatigue, feeling chilled
	Prostatitis
Stomach ache	Wheezing
Irritable bowel	Irritability
Diarrhoea, constipation	Premenstrual tension
Mucus problems anywhere	Dizziness
Muscle aches	Joint pain and swelling
Chronic 'flu symptoms	Burning feet, burning anywhere
Food allergies	
Poor immunity	Severe forgetfulness
Spots before the eyes	Watering eyes

Routine medical tests usually prove negative

- If alcohol really upsets you this can be a strong pointer to candida.

It is not uncommon to find even young people with a long list of symptoms like this. Obviously no one has all of them; they vary considerably. So if you are still mysteriously unwell, especially if you feel you have chronic 'flu or some kind of infection, it could help you a lot to find out more about candida.

Early diagnosis is essential

Candida usually begins in the gut or in the vagina and sometimes appears to confine its worst effects to one or perhaps two systems of the body. This can make it very difficult to recognise from the long and wide-ranging list of symptoms given for chronic candida. So if you have only a few of the symptoms but they are persistent and resistant to medical treatment, it is still worth considering candida. By treating it promptly you could avoid much further trouble.

THE ANTI-CANDIDA DIET

CUT OUT

Sugar	Mushrooms
Yeast	Grapes
Bread	Dried fruit
Yeast extract spreads	Melon
White flour	Peanuts
Cheese	Alcohol
All sweetened foods	Quorn
Any other fermented foods or drinks	

RESTRICT

Fruit	Milk

By keeping strictly to this diet many people experience considerable relief in one to four weeks.

EVERYONE HAS TO DIET.
OTHER TREATMENTS ALONE WILL NOT CURE CANDIDA.

You may already have found that some of these foods upset you or that you take them to excess. Candida bugs have a way of demanding what they like best!

WHY CUT OUT THESE FOODS?

The anti-candida diet is designed to starve the candida.

Sugar and sweetened foods: because candida lives on sugar.
Bread and yeast: because yeast is a fungus.
Mushrooms are also fungi, of course.
White flour turns to sugar in the body.

31

Grapes, dried fruit, melon and any other very ripe fruit are full of sugar and there are invisible natural yeasts on the skins. These can all trigger a flare-up of candida in a very short time.

Quorn is a fungus food.

Peanuts: because they come out of the ground and contain some very nasty moulds.

Fermented foods and drinks are full of yeasts.

Alcohol feeds candida; wine and beer are the worst.

> *Wine:* the yeast on the skin of grapes is what ferments the wine.
>
> *Beer:* Malt is fermented grain.

Cheese of all kinds is also fermented.

Restrict fruit because it contains fructose, which is fruit sugar. All sugar is the same to a candida bug! So make sure any fruit is firm and not over-ripe. Many chronic candida sufferers take fruit to excess; you may have to cut it out competely in order to recover.

Restrict milk because it contains lactose which is milk sugar and does not taste sweet. Soya milk does not contain lactose; make sure it is sugar-free.

Peel root vegetables: there is mould on the skins. Do not eat jacket potato skins.

Leftover food becomes contaminated with yeasts and moulds almost immediately. It causes great problems for some candida sufferers. You could be very surprised how much better you feel without it.

What can I drink?

- Spring water, lemon juice.
- Decaffeinated tea or coffee.
- A little milk.
- Unsweetened soya milk.
- Freshly prepared vegetable juices.

Decaffeinated teabags are available from most supermarkets. They are a compromise of course, as is decaffeinated coffee.

What can I eat instead of bread?

- Potatoes.
- Porridge, rice, millet, barley, quinoa.
- Home-made soda bread.
- Yeast-free crispbreads—plain Ryvita.
- Oatcakes, rice cakes.
- Chapatis.

Be careful: remember that you need plenty of whole grains and potatoes to keep your strength up. Rice cakes and crispbreads are not nearly substantial enough on their own. Low-carbohydrate diets are not a good idea, especially if you suffer from low blood sugar.

Wholewheat flour can still be used in cooking and baking without yeast.

Home-made chapatis: unfortunately most commercial pitta breads, soda breads and Indian flatbreads contain yeast or sugar, so always make your own.

Home-made soda bread is easy to make in batches and can be frozen. Most cookbooks have a recipe for soda bread. If you would miss cakes and biscuits, see Erica White's *Beat Candida Cookbook* (details in Further Reading).

Foods which fight candida

- Garlic is a powerful natural fungicide.
- Natural yoghurt helps candida. It contains the friendly bacteria which fight it.
- Extra virgin olive oil is antifungal.

CHANGE YOUR DIET SLOWLY

Drastic changes in diet can be devastating, especially to someone who is severely affected. Many chronic candida victims also suffer from food intolerance, which is explained in the next chapter, so resist the temptation to rush into your new diet. Take it a step at a time—in any order you like:

1 *Gradually reduce sugar and sweetened food.* Replace it with plenty of whole grains and potatoes. If you crave sugar, carry on with fruit as a temporary measure.
2 *Gradually reduce bread.*
3 *Slowly reduce alcohol.* Try sparkling water with a slice of lemon when you go out.
4 *Gradually replace fruit with raw vegetables and salad:* avocado pears, tomatoes, raw carrots, red and yellow peppers, celery and so on.

KEEP TO THE PRINCIPLES OF THE HAY DIET

Food combining: separating starch from protein reduces bloating and wind.
50 per cent salad and fresh vegetables: if you really cannot take salad, try the raw vegetable soup in Chapter 11. Raw food heals the gut and mucous membrane.

The Hay diet will accelerate your recovery

Many people recover on diet alone

They make good steady progress from the beginning and there is no need for anti-fungal treatment.

SHALL I ALWAYS HAVE TO DIET?
People very according to the strength of their immunity. Some have to keep to the diet very strictly indeed. Others find they can tolerate occasional small lapses. Reactions to forbidden foods can be slow to build up and may not appear for several days, so the connection is not always easy to make.

IS CANDIDA YOUR PROBLEM?

Be careful:
Candida can be a vicious enemy. If you are severely affected you may find that the slightest break in the diet provokes a severe flare-up of symptoms, especially at first. In fact if you *are* very seriously affected, as many people are, it would be safer to get expert nutritional help from the beginning.

VITAMIN AND MINERAL SUPPORT WHILE CHANGING YOUR DIET
Not everybody needs it, but if you feel it would help you could use the programme at the end of the Appendix.

HOW ELSE IS CANDIDA TREATED?

- Vitamins and minerals to rebuild natural resistance to it.
- Evening primrose oil.
- Lactobacillus acidophilus: friendly bacteria which fight candida. Obtainable in capsules from health food shops.
- Caprylic acid, a powerful natural fungicide. Erica White's *Beat Candida Cookbook* contains guidance on taking it.
- Anti-fungal drugs such as Nystatin.

Die-off

When candida is starved it dies off and floods the system with candida toxins. Some people may experience a return of the symptoms for a week or two, until the toxins are eliminated. Not everyone experiences die-off.

Be careful:
Die-off can be severe if you are seriously affected by candida, especially in response to anti-fungal medication, so it is wise to start with a small dose and increase it gradually. In fact it is safer to be professionally supervised while taking it, again by a nutritional therapist or a specialist doctor with experience in treating candida. With expert help you could make a faster recovery.

DRUGS AND CANDIDA

Many people can trace the onset of their illness back to anti-biotics, because they kill off friendly bacteria in the gut which control candida. The risk is greater if they have been taken repeatedly or long term at any time at all during your life.

Other drugs can also increase the tendency to candida

- The contraceptive pill.
- Hormone replacement therapy (HRT).
- Steroid drugs in particular.

Again, this chapter is just a very brief outline intended to help you to recognise candida and to take the first steps in treating it by changing your diet.

CHAPTER 4

Food Intolerance Revealed

It is as well to know about food intolerance before you start on the Hay diet: you need to be aware that, when you do eventually give in to temptation and break the diet after some time without processed food, you may possibly experience a reaction to it. If you are not prepared for this you will be left wondering why you feel unwell and you might think that the Hay diet does not suit you after all.

ALLERGY OR INTOLERANCE?

Food allergy

Most people's understanding of food allergy is that it includes all reactions to food, major and minor, but food allergy as a doctor understands it is actually quite rare. It is the dramatic and unmistakable reaction which some people have to peanuts or to shellfish, for example. This is a well recognised condition with a laboratory test to confirm it.

Food intolerance

In cases of food intolerance reactions are less dramatic and slower to develop—anything from an hour after eating, up to twenty-four hours or more. Usually it involves foods eaten very frequently, so the cause of the trouble is hard to find. Fortunately, however, this is a more treatable condition.

Food intolerance goes largely unrecognised today because, yet again, there is no one hundred-per-cent reliable laboratory test to confirm it. Consequently, as with hypoglycaemia and candida, doctors have no idea that it is so widespread, or that it can cause so many different symptoms and be involved in so many of our common illnesses. However, it has actually been known to medicine for thousands of years. Hippocrates, the father of medicine, was well aware of it centuries before the time of Christ and he identified troublesome foods using methods similar to those described here.

EXPOSING THE PROBLEM

The Hay diet will reveal intolerance of processed foods first of all, usually during the first two or three weeks. Later, often within the first six weeks, you could find that reactions to natural foods like dairy products and wheat will show up. The lists of symptoms given later on will help you to recognise them.

The body struggles bravely to keep us on an even keel each day by suppressing reactions to unsuitable foods, but if the offending foods are excluded for about seven to ten days it relaxes, drops its guard and you begin to feel better. Then, when you try the foods again, it is taken by surprise and you may experience a sharp reaction. Suspect any food you eat to excess or any food which you feel you cannot do without.

Start with the Hay diet

- Cut out all processed foods and replace them with natural foods.
- It works better if you can also separate starch from protein and cut out caffeine.

After about two weeks, or whenever you feel better, re-introduce the processed foods one at a time, in any order you like, as you get tempted, and observe their effects.

THE BIGGEST TROUBLEMAKERS
Sugar and all sweetened foods, especially chocolate, white bread and white flour.

FOOD INTOLERANCE REVEALED

WHAT COULD I EXPECT?
Headaches, tiredness; a 'cold' or 'flu'; stomach pains; any symptoms at all.

Be careful if you are very debilitated
Processed foods can sometimes produce quite severe reactions, so try a small amount at first. However, it is by no means essential to test these foods at all, especially if you are quite happy on natural food.

Asthma? Be extra careful
Food testing may occasionally cause an attack even if you are just a chronic wheezer who rarely gets one, so, again, test with small amounts of food only.

Intolerance of natural foods

Once processed foods have been removed from the diet you become very much more in tune with your body, and if any other food is upsetting you it will let you know. Intolerance of a particular type of food frequently runs in families, often producing different problems in each individual.

ANY FOOD CAN CAUSE A REACTION
The most common offenders are:
- Dairy products, wheat, eggs, peanuts.
- Pork (and bacon and ham).
- Bananas and citrus fruits.

Withdrawal symptoms
If you are taking excessive amounts of any suspect food, withdraw it slowly enough to minimise any discomfort.

INTOLERANCE OF DAIRY PRODUCTS

This is a huge problem. Awareness is definitely growing but still it goes largely unrecognised. Suspect it if you drink a lot of milk or if you eat a lot of cheese. However, not everyone who suffers this way takes dairy products to excess, it can happen to anyone. Cow's milk intolerance is more common in people who were bottle-fed as a baby.

Testing—be very strict or it will not work
For quickest results cut dairy products out entirely, including yoghurt. Some people get symptoms only if they consume more than a certain amount; others may find that it takes only a teaspoonful of milk to cause trouble.

ARE YOU INTOLERANT OF DAIRY PRODUCTS?

These symptoms are typical:

Blocked nose	Anxiety, tension
Ear infections	Nervousness
Sinusitis	Listlessness
Sore throats	Mental fogging
Persistent cough	Lack of confidence
Chest infections	Hyperactivity
Hay fever	Headaches, migraine
Chronic asthma, wheezing	Stomach aches, distension
Frequent infections	Aching legs
Frequent colds	Loose stools
Mucus anywhere	Chronic constipation
Weight gain	Difficulty relaxing for sleep
Joint pains, arthritis	Colitis
Low blood sugar	Low tolerance of stress

What can I drink instead of milk?

Drink water, fruit juice, or herbal teas only—no soya milk, sheep's milk or goat's milk while testing.

- Although some people can take sheep's or goat's milk, others may find they cannot take animal milk of any kind.
- People who are intolerant of milk may also react to soya milk; it can cause bowel problems in particular.
- Rice drinks have recently been introduced but they can be expensive.
- Dietitians can usually help with cutting out dairy products.

FOOD ADDICTION

People who are intolerant of natural foods can actually become addicted to them. Addictions to milk, cheese and chocolate are not uncommon. Cut them down very slowly indeed because withdrawal symptoms can be severe.

What are dairy products?

- Milk of all kinds, cheese, butter, cream, yoghurt.
- Ice-cream, milk chocolate.
- Most margarines contain milk.

There is milk in processed foods of many kinds and in various baked goods, including some bread, but you may not have to worry about small amounts unless you are very sensitive.

- Hard cheese usually causes the most trouble.
- Eggs are not dairy products, but they are another common cause of allergy, especially egg whites.

What about calcium?

On an all-natural diet we can easily obtain enough calcium for our needs from natural foods, including:

- Green leafy vegetables, whole grains, eggs.
- Fruit, especially dried fruit.
- Nuts, seeds, beans.
- Fish, especially those, like sardines, which have edible bones.
- Tahini (sesame seed spread) and tofu (soya cheese).

CALCIUM ROBBERS

Sugar, sweetened foods and soft drinks, especially cola, all rob us of calcium; so by cutting them out you retain more of it.

INTOLERANCE OF GLUTEN

This is another very common cause of trouble which is rarely recognised. Gluten is the protein part of wheat, rye, barley and oats, and any products containing these may cause an adverse reaction.

Where do I find gluten?

- Wheat and wheat products: bread, pasta, semolina; bulgur wheat, cracked wheat.
- Oatmeal, porridge.
- Rye crispbreads, barley.
- Rye bread may also contain wheat.

What can I eat instead?

- Jacket potatoes.
- Gluten-free whole grains: sweet corn and maize; brown rice, millet, quinoa, raw buckwheat.

What about tapioca and sago?

Although they are both gluten-free they are not whole and balanced foods like grains, so their nutritional value is much lower, just as it is in white rice and the refined flours.

ARE YOU INTOLERANT OF GLUTEN?

It can cause:

Bloating, wind	Chronic tiredness
Stomach aches	Nervous stomach
Abdominal distension	Chronic constipation
Indigestion, acidity	Morning stupor
Irritability	Aggression
Loose stools	Sleeping problems
Hay fever	Wheezing, asthma
Irritable bowel	Nightmares
Joint pains, arthritis	Mood swings
Headaches, migraine	Depression
Gnawing hunger	Stress problems

Severe cravings for wheat; nothing else will do

- Tapioca comes from the cassava or manioc root.
- Sago is prepared from the starchy pith underneath the bark of the sago palm.

More information on the other grains can be found in Chapter 11.

Food testing

Many people who have problems with wheat are also affected by the other gluten grains, but not everybody. Remember to cut down slowly if you eat lots of bread.

- Keep all gluten grains out of the diet for up to a month, or until you feel better, because grains are very slowly absorbed. Gluten can take up to three weeks to leave the system completely, so you may not feel better straight away.
- Re-introduce gluten grains one by one, and wait for any symptoms to clear before trying another. Meanwhile be sure

to eat plenty of the other non-gluten grains while testing, to keep up your blood sugar level.

Some of us are intolerant of the gluten-free grains too, although rice is well tolerated by most people.

Digestive enzymes have been found to help some people who suffer from food intolerance. They can be useful in situations where you cannot avoid problem foods. They are taken with the food:

> *Prolactazyme Forte* for dairy products. It covers lactose, milk protein and milk fats.
> *Glutenzyme* helps to digest gluten.
> *Broad spectrum digestive enzymes* can help with a range of other foods.

Suppliers are listed under 'Useful Addresses'

SHALL I ALWAYS BE INTOLERANT OF FOOD?
After a period of avoidance some people find that they lose their intolerance. If it is stubborn you may find that as natural healing progresses you may gradually become less sensitive.

MULTIPLE FOOD INTOLERANCES

The Hay diet can expose a limited number of food intolerances only. If you are very debilitated and have many problems it will be just the first step in the right direction. The way forward is to keep strictly to natural foods and to investigate the underlying causes with professional help from a doctor who specialises in nutritional medicine.

Neutralising injections can work very well, although people vary in their response to them. They are definitely not the incremental desensitising injections which were discontinued a few years ago for safety reasons. Dr John Mansfield has been using this treatment for many years and discusses it in his book *The Migraine Revolution*.

Make sure you get skilled help with managing a very restricted diet as not all doctors currently working in nutritional medicine work with a dietitian or a nutritional therapist. See Useful Addresses at the end of this book for more information.

Having read this far you may be thinking . . .

But these lists of symptoms could apply to almost any illness, couldn't they?
True, but there is a pattern in them which a sufferer will usually recognise; if you are well you will not see it.

Everyone has symptoms like this from time to time, don't they?
Yes, but it is only the persistent symptoms that really count— those which crop up all too frequently.

CHAPTER 5

Food Combining

Whether you keep to the Hay diet long term and adopt it as your way of life will depend on how much you understand it, so make the changes one at a time as your understanding grows. A small change firmly fitted into your life is often a more lasting one. Changing too quickly may make you miserable and force you to abandon the regime altogether, but the experience can teach you a lot—you may well discover a very good reason for keeping to the Hay diet in future.

DON'T MIX FOODS THAT FIGHT!

Concentrated proteins
Meat, fish, eggs and cheese
are separated from . . .

Concentrated starches
Potatoes and grains
plus
Sugar and all sweetened foods**

They are eaten at separate meals:
either a starch-based meal or a protein-based meal

Learn to separate these foods first. It takes a long time and many mistakes. It may be weeks or even months before food combining becomes second nature.

Vegetables except potatoes go with any meal.
Salad of all kinds goes with any meal.
**Aim to cut out sugar and all sweetened foods eventually.

Don't Mix Foods That Fight!

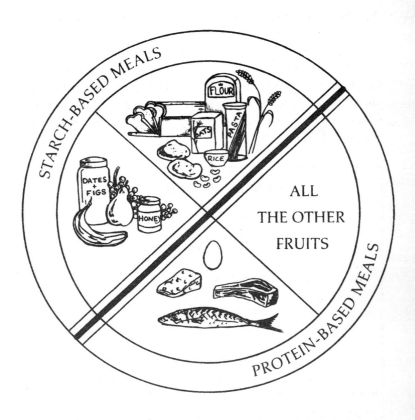

Changing the habits of a lifetime

As each new change becomes a habit you will feel more able to cope with another; it requires much patience. The occasional treat will do no harm—it's what you eat all the time that counts. But be careful if you are very debilitated: you could get an unpleasant reaction from incompatible mixtures of food once you have been in the habit of food combining for some time.

Why do books on food combining differ so much?
Food combining is nothing new, we are just rediscovering an ancient principle. There are actually several other systems of food combining and even books on the Hay diet differ in many ways, according to the convictions of the writer. Of course people like to know where they are and it would be a lot easier if the same set of rules could apply to everyone, but the human body is not like that—we are individuals. So just listen to your body and go along with whatever helps most.

How long between a starch meal and a protein meal?

Ideally three to four hours. The main digestion of starch takes place in the first 30 to 45 minutes.

Protein takes two to four hours to digest. It spends much longer in the stomach because it is digested there.

Can I have extra meals?

Yes of course!

Snacks between meals have become a way of life for many of us, mainly because of low blood sugar. Many people find that they can reduce the time between starch and protein meals without ill-effects provided they do not actually eat the starch and protein together.

How much food?

Most people find that they need less to eat on the Hay diet because food is better absorbed. Smaller meals actually release a lot more energy, so have enough for your present need and no more.

A SIMPLE REMEDY

Proper food combining can be a tremendous relief to the digestive system; the list of symptoms below shows just how much strain we can put on it by combining foods badly. After a couple of weeks on food combining most people find that they prefer to eat this way— their stomach objects if they don't! The motivation to continue on the diet comes from the relief it gives, and those who benefit from it usually find that if they lapse, the symptoms return.

FOOD COMBINING
This has been the experience of many people

RELIEF FROM:

Afternoon sluggishness	Sleeping after meals
Blocked or runny nose	Belching, bloating, wind
Indigestion	Sinusitis
Heartburn	Wheezing, asthma
Constipation	Eczema
Joint pains	Allergies
Swollen feet	Irritable bowel
Low blood sugar	Morning sickness

How long before I get results?

Some people respond astonishingly quickly, especially if they are reasonably fit anyway. Digestive problems and minor allergies can clear up within days; long-standing problems like asthma, eczema and arthritis will take longer but will still show considerable improvement.

Food combining alone!

I'm not dieting, just food combining, and I've lost a stone. The bloating went straight away, my stomach went right down.

I've always had a healthy diet, but since I've been separating the foods I feel great; my skin is softer and my hair is growing again.

I use food combining to keep my weight down; I have two days off it every week.

Food combining is the only thing that helps. My energy goes up, my digestion improves, everything comes together; but if I mix the foods it all comes back. Once you get beyond a certain age you just feel better separating starch from protein.

My itchy eyes and runny nose cleared up immediately.

My bowels are working really well at last, but if I mix the starch and the protein I get constipated again.

I'm only separating the foods. It's hard work but I've managed to reduce my anti-anxiety tablets, so something must be happening.

The effect of food combining is more than doubled when you cut out processed food altogether and substitute natural food with plenty of fresh fruit, raw vegetables and salad.

WHY SEPARATE STARCH FROM PROTEIN?

What happens to starch?

Starch digestion is alkaline and it begins in the mouth; with thorough chewing the saliva begins to turn the starch to sugar. Saliva is alkaline and when the food reaches the stomach it carries on with the job of digesting the starch; there is not enough gastric acid to interfere with its work, provided we do not eat concentrated protein with it. The stomach just churns the food around, gradually releasing it into the small intestine where the main digestion of starch takes place.

What happens to protein?

Protein is digested in acid. When concentrated protein enters the stomach it triggers the release of just the right amount of gastric acid required to break it down.

What happens when we eat starch and protein together?

This is the theory:

- The stomach contents are neutralised and incompletely digested foods can then ferment in the digestive system, leading to bloating, belching and wind.
- Large molecules of incompletely digested protein, including histamine, can then enter the bloodstream, causing allergic reactions of all kinds.
- Emptying of the stomach is delayed, often leading to constipation.

But surely grains and many of the vegetables contain starch and protein together, so why don't they cause any trouble? Because no natural food actually contains both *concentrated* starch and *concentrated* protein together; either starch or protein predominates. Grains, for example, are mainly starch with very little protein, not enough to interfere with digestion; and of course meat is high in protein.

WHAT IS WRONG WITH THESE COMBINATIONS?	
Cheese pizza	Cheese quiche
Shepherd's pie	Meat curry with rice
Pasta with cheese sauce	Fish and chips
Beefburger in a roll	Apple pie
Roast beef and roast potatoes	Cheese sandwich
Egg on toast	Meat pie
Cheese on toast	Beefburger in a roll
Egg sandwich	Meat sandwich

What about dried beans or peas?
Once they are soaked, the proportions of starch and protein return to normal—that is, they are mostly starch and water with

about five per cent protein. The principles of food combining obey the laws of nature.

THIS IS A MORE NATURAL WAY TO EAT

Our ancestors who lived in the forest were hunter-gatherers; they picked berries, they dug up starchy roots and they hunted animals for meat; they would probably have eaten most of their foods one at a time.

WHAT ABOUT FRUIT?

Eating fruit with meals is no problem to the majority of people if they follow Dr Hay's method of food combining:

With starch-based meals: bananas, yellow pears, grapes, dates and figs.
With protein-based meals: all the other fruits.

Some books based on food combining follow the teachings of the American Natural Hygiene Movement. These differ from the Hay diet in that fruit is never eaten with meals; it is taken mainly in the morning on an empty stomach. Sometimes people who believe they cannot take fruit find to their delight that it causes no trouble if they eat it on its own.

IF FOOD COMBINING DOES NOT APPEAR TO HELP

Carry on with it; a complete change to natural food solves a lot more problems. The worse the problem, the more strictly you need to keep to an all-natural diet. Most people enjoy food combining; their strength and stamina improve and they never want to return to the old way of eating. But occasionally, very active people or those with a heavy job may begin to lose their vitality after some time on food combining. They find it imposs-ible to get enough starch to fuel their energy and are forced to abandon it.

A few others are never really happy on it; they just cannot adapt to it however hard they try. So don't make yourself miserable: if you *must* have potatoes with your meat, just concentrate on changing over to an all-natural diet and you will still benefit enormously.

LOSE WEIGHT BY FOOD COMBINING

If you are already on a natural diet but still cannot lose weight, the Hay diet could well be the answer; many people find that it works where all else has failed. Dr Hay once put forty men on an identical diet of healthy food for three months. Half 'did not mix foods that fight', and all of these lost a considerable amount of weight without extra exercise. The others combined their starch and protein in the usual way and lost no weight at all.

Are you losing too much weight?

Slimmers are delighted at first when they lose weight so easily on the Hay diet, but sometimes it continues to drop. People who diet for health reasons can sometimes lose more weight than they intended, so watch your weight very carefully, especially if you are not well; you can prevent any drastic weight loss.

Too thin?

Sometimes, after an initial loss, the weight does stabilise or return to normal because food is better absorbed, but if you are not well your body could be so preoccupied with essential repairs that it may be some considerable time before it can adjust your weight—up or down. If you continue to lose, do make sure that you really are having enough to eat, because if you are to gain weight you must have nutrients to spare. You will need to learn more about nutrition and how to balance your diet. There is more information in Chapter 8.

CHAPTER 6

How Toxic Are You?

Food combining seems to have become the hallmark of the Hay diet in recent years, but separating starch from protein is really only the first step; there are two entirely separate principles involved. The second and most important step is to cut out processed food and replace it with natural food. A simple diet like this would have been quite normal to us a hundred and fifty years ago, but nowadays highly processed convenience foods have become so much a part of our lives that a change to natural food can be very unwelcome at first; it is a hard lesson to learn.

We are rightly concerned about the risks of too many chemical additives, yet we are surprisingly indifferent to what is being taken out of our food. We still buy packaged foods however highly processed they are, provided there are no chemical additives mentioned on the label, but foods like this are dead, deficient; they drain our vitality. They have had the living ingredients processed out of them to prevent them from going bad in the shops. The refining of food, particularly carbohydrates like sugar and white flour, can have extremely toxic and damaging effects on the body, especially in the long term. The recent outbreak of BSE, mad cow disease, is a sharp reminder of how dangerous it can be to interfere with nature's way of feeding.

The symptoms listed in the box (p. 55) are all possible indications of toxicity, due largely to the slow and insidious effects of processed foods, additives and pesticides as they gradually build up in the body. Their effect is imperceptible, as it is with tobacco, which adds to the problem. This is where degeneration begins: even the fittest-looking person will admit to a health problem of some kind these days.

HOW DO YOU FEEL?

Tired

Low energy

Irritable, grumpy

Aches and pains

No smile

Stiff joints

Run down

Poor immunity

Frequent colds and infections

Feeling unwell at times

A grey, toxic complexion
   (washing makes no difference)

Bored

Headaches

Forgetful

Few ideas

Unaware

Unhappy

Poor concentration

Easily stressed

Tense

Nervous

A poor diet upsets the delicate balance of nature; it disrupts body chemistry and disturbs our blood sugar balance. We develop hormone imbalances: things just don't work together properly any more. It accelerates ageing and sets us on the road to degenerative illness. It can take many years for the full effects of a bad diet to appear, but it catches up with most of us eventually. The more unnatural our diet, the sooner we suffer.

DEGENERATIVE DISEASE

This is the result of long-term mental and physical deterioration and it includes:

Cancer

Strokes

Heart attacks

High blood pressure

High blood cholesterol

Arthritis

Chronic asthma

Peptic ulcers

Chronic mental illness

Alzheimer's disease

Skin disease

Kidney disease

These are the foods that harm

They are toxic when taken to excess. They are all junk foods.

- Sugar and all sweetened foods:
    Biscuits, cakes, chocolate, ice-cream.
- Soft drinks.
- White bread and white flour.
- Potato crisps, salted snacks.
- Margarine and ordinary processed cooking oil.
- Any other highly processed artificial foods.

Junk food can be powerfully addictive and some of us are much more susceptible to it than others. The trouble is that, once we get the taste for food that is artificially concentrated and flavoured with sugar, salt and other additives, we can no longer rely on our natural instincts to tell us what is good for us, we just want more of it. We may even come to dislike fresh fruit and salad altogether, finding it bland and uninteresting by comparison. We may reach the point where we want little else to eat but junk food, and this can be a great problem, especially amongst children and young people; they lack vitality and often they are far from well.

However, an all-natural diet soon puts us back in tune with our body and its needs, and children in particular can become very much calmer and easier to manage. Mercifully, the body can regenerate itself at any age—it's never too late—and this is where the Hay diet comes in. Natural healing is marvellous: you just go on from strength to strength, year after year.

This is how we deteriorate

We can only function efficiently so long as we can keep the blood clear of the waste products produced by our own body cells each day. Natural food burns cleanly in the body; it leaves very little waste because it comes with enough vitamins and minerals to digest and absorb it completely. Food processing strips away many of these nutrients, forcing us to take them from body stores—white sugar, for example, contains no vitamins or minerals whatsoever. We cannot handle food like this, not in the large amounts many people eat today. It progressively depletes our vitamin and mineral reserves and, as the years go by, we may become increasingly run down and accumulate a growing number of symptoms.

ARE YOU OVERLOADING YOUR LIVER?

Our liver is only designed to cleanse us of the limited amount of debris produced by natural food. Junk food creates an excessive amount of waste and can place such an unnatural load on the liver that it has to call on other systems of the body to help get rid of it. It uses every possible means to keep us well.

Other means of elimination are:
- *Through the skin:* greasy skin, greasy hair, sweat, body odour, eczema, pimples, acne, boils.
- *Through the kidneys:* in the urine.
- *Through the lungs:* bad breath, cough, phlegm.
- *Through the mucous membranes:* colds, catarrh.
- *Through the bowel.*

Symptoms like these indicate that the body has a battle on its hands and that it needs our assistance.

AFTER THE FEAST COMES THE RECKONING!

The level of toxicity in our bodies is changing all the time and when it gets too much we become unwell. A familiar example is what so often happens after Christmas, when the toxic build-up from too much rich food lowers our resistance to such an extent that whole families go down with infections.

TOXIC ACID BUILD-UP

Some of us are more affected by junk food than others. It largely depends on how effectively our liver and the other systems of elimination are able to detoxify us. Some of us inherit a very much more efficient system than others. Unless we can detoxify ourselves daily, toxic waste gradually builds up in the system over the years and is deposited around the body in much the same way that coke clogs an engine:

- It circulates in the blood, clouding the mind and making us tired and run down, sluggish and bad-tempered.
- It can accumulate in the arteries and in the joints.
- Overeating increases the toxic load because we can only absorb a certain amount of food at one meal. The rest turns to acid waste.
- Incompatible mixtures of food can also increase toxicity because the food is not completely digested.
- When we are under stress all body functions slow down, including toxin elimination.
- A chronically sick person is saturated with acid waste.

Toxic fat

Additives, pesticides and toxic acid residues are frequently stored out of harm's way, in body fat, where they saturate the tissues, leading to cellulite. This means that as you detoxify the fat will often disappear too—another reason why people can lose weight so easily on the Hay diet.

One man's meat is another man's poison

If you are intolerant of any natural food the body treats that as toxic too and, again, it may store it in fat. People with food intolerances are often mysteriously overweight despite a normal appetite and a healthy diet, but the pounds can melt away once any problem foods are identified and excluded.

Chronic constipation is toxic too

A constipated bowel can make you feel very tired and unwell, but clearing it brings a surprising improvement. An overloaded bowel is like a clogged drain, it is another major cause of ill-health. In the long term it can contribute to varicose veins, haemorrhoids (piles), diverticulitis and bowel cancer. Many people experience relief from chronic constipation on the Hay diet. As muscle tone returns to the body as a whole the bowel very gradually recovers; the important thing is to keep it clear in the meantime.

TERRIFYING EPIDEMICS

Cancer, strokes and heart attacks have been building up for a very long time before they strike, but the body will still fight back if we give it the opportunity. Every death from cancer and heart disease is premature; people who have worked hard and taken care of themselves as well as they know how are having their lives cut tragically short.

Hospices are opening at an alarming rate and more younger people than ever are being admitted. The trend will continue unless we change our diet and lifestyle. Dr Hay realised that much cancer is the result of long-standing internal pollution. Removing the tumour can be a life-saving measure, but operations alone do not deal with the underlying toxicity. That is up to us. A positive approach is powerfully therapeutic.

Nature has ways of dealing with cancer too

The Hay diet is a low-risk diet; if you are recovering from cancer it enables you to regain your strength more quickly and reduces the chance of a recurrence. It helps the body to detoxify. Fresh fruit and vegetable juices especially are extremely powerful in this respect; they are central to the natural treatment of cancer. Very gradually, as general health improves, tumours have been known to regress, to dissolve or to encapsulate naturally. By correcting deficiencies of vitamins, minerals and essential fatty acids you can further re-arm your natural defences. Powerful non-toxic homoeopathic and herbal remedies are also available.

Of course, there is a point of no return, but natural treatments have produced some surprising results. Much depends on your vitality and your natural healing capacity. Even in advanced illness natural treatments can bring great relief and are wonderfully soothing. Dr Jan De Vries enlarges on this in *Cancer and Leukaemia: An Alternative Approach*. He has long experience of treating cancer naturally.

Quantum leaps in medical understanding

The work of Dr John Tilden (1851-1940) also makes fascinating reading because he too discovered natural medicine after practising orthodox medicine for many years. He found that he was able to treat most people effectively without drugs and without surgery, mainly by detoxifying the body.

Dr Hay, a surgeon himself, only ever had to send three people to a surgeon in over twenty years once he understood how to treat them naturally. He realised that 'we are born with an imperfect heredity and we build on it a toxic state that grows deeper year by year'. He spoke a different language from that of conventional medicine. The Hay diet gives us a new and more helpful understanding of our body. Symptoms are taken together as a warning that we are treating ourselves badly and need to make some changes.

CHAPTER 7

The Essentials of a Healthy Diet

A well-balanced diet consisting entirely of natural whole foods is actually the only healthy diet there is, but you have to experience it to believe it. A few weeks on the Hay diet are enough to convince most people: it very soon reveals just how much processed food affects us from day to day and how much it slows us down. Replacing it with fresh food vastly increases our intake of vitamins and minerals, and this is what can bring such a rapid and powerful improvement.

The brain is the first part of the body to respond to a clean supply of blood and intellectual performance can improve substantially—we limit our mental capacity through the wrong choice of food. People whose health has never been very good may find that by keeping processed foods permanently out of their diet they function better than ever before; the rewards are immense.

We need at least 50 per cent raw food

At least half your food intake should consist of fresh fruit, salad and raw vegetables. Always cook grains, meat and fish. The salad habit can be difficult to acquire, especially if you are not well, but the lift you get encourages you to carry on. Raw foods contain enzymes which are destroyed by cooking; they break the food down ready for absorption into the body. We can make our own enzymes, but for efficient digestion we do need the extra help from raw food.

WHAT WILL RAW FOOD DO FOR ME?	
Cleanse	Improve mental function
Invigorate	Speed healing
Improve digestion	Relieve stress
Lift depression	Clear your skin
Calm the mind	Improve stamina
Regenerate the body	Clear your head
Strengthen immunity	Condition your hair
Delay ageing	Assist recovery

After a few days without any sugar at all in the diet, your taste buds wake up to the fresh and exciting flavours of natural food. You very soon come to prefer the scent and flavour of fresh fruit, and all the colour and variety of a crisp salad.

ACID AND ALKALINE

Acid and alkaline are not the foods that fight, they mix quite happily together. These terms describe the effect of foods on the blood after they have been digested and absorbed in the body. Alkalinity of body tissues means a good state of health and a strong resistance to disease, but an over-acid system leads to debility and sickness. So far this theory has received little support from conventional nutrition because, like food combining, it is not yet fully understood, but it too works extremely well in practice. It is central to an understanding of the Hay diet.

Alkali-forming foods

These foods leave behind a highly beneficial alkaline deposit, a mineral ash. The alkaline reserve is the store of alkali-forming minerals, kept ready to neutralise the acid waste produced naturally by body cells as they go about their work each day.

They keep the system clean and play a vital role in maintaining natural immunity.

Alkali-forming foods are:
- Salad and vegetables.
- Millet and jacket potatoes.
- Most fruits, including dried fruit.

But how can acid fruits be alkali-forming?

'Acid' fruit just means that these fruits need acid digestion, like protein. The acid they contain leaves the body within an hour, mostly via the lungs, and the remaining alkaline minerals are deposited in the system and kept in reserve.

- The more acid-tasting a fruit is, the more alkali-forming it will be. Citrus fruits, especially lemons, are richest in minerals.
- Some truly acid-forming exceptions are plums, rhubarb and cranberries, which are not strictly recommended.

Fats and oils are neutral, neither acid-forming nor alkali-forming.

ALKALI-FORMING MINERALS

Potassium, calcium, magnesium

Where are they found?
In natural foods of all kinds
especially fresh fruit and vegetables.
The small amounts of sodium found naturally in whole
foods are also alkali-forming.

Let your food be your medicine
We absorb vitamins and minerals best from natural food.

Freshly prepared fruit or vegetable juices are a refreshing and powerful natural tonic, full of alkali-forming minerals. The effect of just one drink, straight from an electric juicer, may well be enough to convince you; the lift can be almost immediate. Carry on with them for faster results.

Getting the balance right

Since food technology developed and since we have become so much more affluent, the balance of our diet has gradually changed from alkaline to acid, due mainly to the over-consumption of heavily processed foods like sugar and white flour. This is a degenerative diet; it creates health problems of every kind.

Why do we have to know which foods are acid-forming?
Because nowadays so many of us are eating up to eighty per cent acid-forming food when it should actually be the other way round; we need nearer eighty per cent alkali-forming food if we are to avoid illness or to recover our health.

Acid-forming foods

Natural acid-forming foods are nevertheless vital to the body. We must have adequate protein for body maintenance and repair and we must also eat enough carbohydrate for warmth, energy and optimum mental functioning. We are naturally designed to eat limited amounts of these foods and to clear ourselves daily of the debris they produce.

These are healthy acid-forming foods:
- Grains except millet.
- Meat, fish, eggs, cheese.
- Dried beans, peas and lentils.

Concentrated proteins

Meat, fish, cheese and eggs are strongly acid-forming; they are by far the most acid-producing foods of all so they have to be taken in strict moderation.

High-protein diets

Too much animal protein, especially meat, places by far the heaviest burden on the digestive system; the body has to work extremely hard to neutralise it. Too much protein will overload the kidneys because the acids it produces have to be passed out in the urine. So if you already lack vitality, a high-protein diet will add to the problem.

Concentrated starches

- The waste products from carbohydrate foods are mainly water, and carbon dioxide which is excreted by the lungs.
- Natural carbohydrates such as jacket potatoes and whole grains produce far less acid than protein foods.
- Wheat and rye are more acid-forming than the other grains.

Pulses: Beans, peas and lentils create more acid than any of the grains.

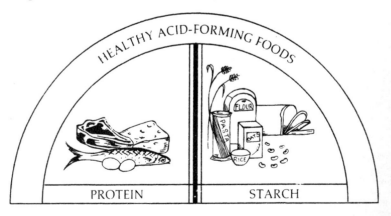

HEALTHY ACID-FORMING FOODS

PROTEIN   STARCH

ACID-FORMING MINERALS ARE ALSO VITAL TO THE BODY

Sulphur, phosphorus, chloride

Where are they found?
In balanced amounts in natural foods.
They only cause trouble if we take them to excess.
Sulphur helps to form sulphuric acid.
Phosphorus helps to form phosphoric acid.
Chloride helps to make hydrochloric acid (stomach acid).

Sodium chloride is common salt
Too much salt is acid-forming because it attracts acid into body cells. Sulphates, phosphates and sodium compounds are used very extensively in food processing. In his book *E for Additives* Maurice Hanssen reveals the astonishing extent of it.

CHANGING OVER TO NATURAL FOOD

Most people feel better within a day or two of changing over to an all-natural diet, but it is possible that you may feel worse for a time after the initial lift, for several reasons:

- You could be changing your diet too quickly. Stored toxins are released into the bloodstream as you detoxify, and you may be releasing them faster than you can eliminate them. Raw vegetables and salad detoxify more slowly and more gently than fruit.
- You may be experiencing withdrawal symptoms from foods to which you are unknowingly intolerant.

What can you expect?
Headaches, depression, sleeping problems, aches and pains, any symptoms at all. Carry on with the Hay diet, it should pass if you

are reasonably fit. If you continue to feel unwell there may be other reasons for this, including low blood sugar.

Restoring the balance

The aim of the Hay diet is to change the balance of our diet from acid back to alkaline as nature intended. Fresh fruit and vegetables, alkali-forming foods high in potassium, made up most of the diet of early humans. These are the foods on which we developed and they are the most natural to the human body. Acid-forming foods like meat and grains were in short supply. The Hay diet follows this same natural pattern of eating. Every natural food is perfectly balanced and on an all-natural diet this natural balance is reflected in us, in a sane mind and a healthy body.

CHAPTER 8

Adapt the Hay Diet to Your Own Needs

The Hay diet provides a perfect balance for many people, but obviously no one set of rules can suit everybody. If you feel unwell on it or if you have been ill for a long time, you will need to learn more about food and the way it is affecting you. Most people feel that their diet is good and it can be quite a shock to find out just how unbalanced and how far from ideal it really is. Often you can see straight away why you feel so unwell and why you are taking so long to recover. Getting it right gives you a tremendous boost and the improvement goes on and on.

Very often weak and debilitated people are not actually having enough to eat, so just increasing the amounts of food could be enough to revive you considerably. You may need to alter the amounts of starch and protein; the quantities needed will depend on how efficiently you digest and absorb your food. You can usually find out what is right for you by experiment, being guided by the way you feel.

A diet restricted by food intolerances or candida needs careful checking. If you have a long list of problem foods you must know exactly what to eat instead, preferably before you begin, because a very unbalanced diet only leads to more problems. A dietitian or a nutritional therapist could check it for you.

WATER WORKS WONDERS

Are you drinking enough? We need about a litre of
fluid a day.

What will water do for me?

Increase energy

Improve digestion

Lessen food cravings

Moisturise your skin

Ease bladder problems

Flush out toxins

Relieve tension

Clear your head

Ease constipation

Improve cellulite

Reduce fluid retention

Speed healing

When do I drink it?

- Between meals.
- Half an hour before a meal.
- Or sip it gradually over the day.
- If you wake up thirsty during the night, it helps to drink more during the day.
- Drinking large amounts with meals dilutes the digestive juices and can lead to indigestion.

If you only drink when you are thirsty you may not get enough fluid. If you are not drinking very much water you will be surprised at how much fresher and cleaner you feel if you drink more. It can be hard at first, but if you persevere you will soon feel the benefit.

Once you get into the habit of drinking more water you will find that your body demands it, so listen to your body and be sure to drink whenever you feel thirsty. Every cell in the body needs a clean supply of water to carry out its work properly, so it makes sense to keep it moving. Stagnation allows body waste to accumulate in the tissues. The human body is approximately sixty per cent water.

Be careful: If you drink too much water, food will pass through the system too quickly, before it can be properly absorbed.

ARE YOU DEHYDRATED?

Lots of people are dehydrated without realising it, often without feeling particularly thirsty. If you can pinch up the skin on your forearm and it does not immediately spring back flat again, then you must be somewhat dehydrated. A little more water may even iron out a few wrinkles!

Tea and coffee are dehydrating

The caffeine they contain is a diuretic, it makes us pass more urine; so if you rely on them too much you will pass more fluid than you are taking in.

Tap water can make you tired

The chemicals in tap water may affect sensitive people; they can also cause eczema, bowel problems—any symptoms at all. You could be very surprised indeed at the difference pure spring water can make: energy levels have been known to improve very considerably and stubborn symptoms can often disappear.

Fresh fruit and vegetables and their juices

Fresh fruit and vegetables have a high water content, and the water they contain is laden with vitamins and minerals in the form the body most prefers. Eat them whole if you can, but if you are unwell it is worth going to the trouble of making juices.

- Juices work best if you drink them straight away but they can be frozen for a few hours. If you add a teaspoonful of extra virgin olive oil it will help with the absorption of the fat-soluble vitamins (A and E).
- The raw vegetable soup on page 113 can be used instead of juices.

ARE YOU GETTING ENOUGH CARBOHYDRATE?

Or are you running out of fuel?

Signs of carbohydrate deficiency

Constant worrying
Cold hands and feet
Sleeping problems
Depression
Poor concentration
Sudden tiredness: 'running out of steam'
Hungry, tired, sluggish

Seeing everything in a bad light
Muscles tire easily
Difficulty coping
Nervous tension
Indecision, confusion
Panic over little things
Difficulty keeping warm

These problems are all too familiar to slimmers, of course, especially during the first two or three weeks of a diet, and unless you are careful it can happen on the Hay diet too. Again these are symptoms of low blood sugar. They are preventable and easily remedied once you understand what is going on.

Our glycogen (starch) reserves are kept in the liver and in the muscles and we only store about 1,000–2,000 calories, enough for 24–48 hours. Slimmers frequently run their reserves right down because they know so little about low blood sugar, and the resulting exhaustion and muscle weakness can be devastating. We need to eat regularly in order to maintain our reserves, so that we have enough to keep us feeling well and to sustain us whenever we need a quick burst of energy.

You will soon get to know when your reserves are running low because the tension and tiredness come back. By increasing your intake of complex carbohydrates you could well feel calmer, more relaxed and stronger physically; it can sometimes take several days to replenish yourself. You will be surprised and intrigued at how much you can improve your energy and your state of mind; some people recover astonishingly quickly.

One starch meal a day suits many Hay-dieters, but a very active person, or someone whose job is physically demanding,

---

HOW MUCH CARBOHYDRATE DO I NEED?

Up to four or five servings
of concentrated starch per day
plus
five pieces of fresh fruit
(about 500 g or one pound)
Carbohydrate includes both concentrated starch foods
and the natural sugars in whole fruits because starch
turns to sugar in the body.
Dietitians recommend 50 per cent of calories as
natural carbohydrate

---

usually needs more than one starch meal a day to fuel his or her energy. Children too need more carbohydrate.

Don't forget to maintain your alkaline balance
Jacket potatoes and millet are alkali-forming, but wholemeal bread, peeled potatoes, brown rice and porridge are all acid-forming, so balance each meal with plenty of salad. A starch meal taken with oil or butter is more sustaining because fat delays emptying of the stomach.

ARE YOU GETTING ENOUGH PROTEIN?

Lack of protein can cause:

Poor hair and nail growth
Dry, unmanageable hair
Dry, flaking skin
Cracked heels and fingertips
Wrinkles, premature ageing
Constant hunger
Fluid retention
Frequent infections

Fatigue, low energy
Poor memory
Poor concentration
Mood problems
Poor muscle tone
Weak, soft muscles
Poor posture
Constipation

Many of us go short of protein because we do not know enough about food; we store very little protein so we must have some every day. It is a basic body-building material and part of the structure of every cell in the body. We need it for running repairs, to make the digestive enzymes which break down the food, and for making blood cells, especially the white cells which fight infection. So never miss a protein meal—lack of it causes havoc throughout the body and always leads to illness.

Having a good protein-based meal every single day can make a surprising difference to the way you feel. If you lack energy and concentration you could well feel physically stronger and much more alert.

HOW MUCH PROTEIN DO I NEED?

50–100 g (two to four ounces)
concentrated protein a day
Meat ● Fish ● Cheese ● Eggs

Individual protein needs vary considerably and some people manage to keep fit and well on less than the recommended amount. Not everyone can be a vegetarian: meat and fish are essential to some of us.

- Salad eaten with concentrated protein provides extra vitamins and minerals to aid digestion and to neutralise its acidity.
- Mysteriously persistent difficulty with digesting protein can sometimes be due to the effects of low blood sugar, caused by insufficient concentrated starch in the diet.

Too much animal protein

We do not need nearly as much protein as was once thought. Animal protein foods are not whole foods; they are not balanced foods in the way that whole plant foods like grains are. The digestion of animal protein, especially meat, is therefore depleting. In order to digest it fully the body is forced to draw the missing vitamins and minerals from body stores, especially calcium and some of the B vitamins. Again, it is this continual drain on our reserves which contributes to a progressive deterioration in our mental and physical condition.

Vegetable protein in starch meals

On the Hay diet, at least one third of our daily protein requirement will come from plant sources and, as you can see, natural vegetable proteins are much easier to digest. Other good sources of vegetable protein include nuts and seeds, peas, beans and avocado pears.

ARE YOU SHORT OF ESSENTIAL OILS?

These are common symptoms of deficiency:

Dry, pimply skin	Hormone problems, PMT
Acne, blackheads	Greasy hair
Eczema, rough skin	Depression
Slow healing	Mental problems
Falling hair	Anxiety, panics
Dry mouth, thirst	Allergies
Sore, bleeding gums	Hyperactivity
Digestive problems	Irritability
Bowel problems	Sleeping problems
Nerve pains	Low body temperature
Breast pain	Dry eyes
Poor immunity	Stiff joints
Lack of energy	

Essential fats form part of every cell in the body, so you can see how a lack of them can cause so many problems.

This deficiency has become a major cause of ill-health nowadays because so many of us have been following low-fat diets for a long time, not knowing that we actually need certain fats. These essential fats are found in natural, unprocessed foods.

- They form approximately 30 per cent of the brain.
- They make up the sheaths of all our nerves.
- They help to make and regulate hormones.
- They soften the skin and put a shine on our hair.
- We use them for fuel, for warmth and for energy.

The essential fatty acids they contain are not actually acid-forming.

How do we become so deficient?

Low-fat diets
Anti-candida diets
Restricted allergy diets
Too much of the wrong kinds of fat

All the above can contribute to a deficiency of essential oils. Low-fat diets are intended to reduce only the unhealthy fats, those which contribute to weight gain and degenerative illness. Extra virgin olive oil and foods which are naturally rich in essential fats and oils are still as necessary to people on a low-fat diet as they are to everyone else. You may be surprised to learn that all the essential fats and oils are cholesterol-free.

The absorption of essential oils is blocked by:

- Too much sugar and sweetened food.
- Too much saturated animal fat, especially meat and dairy products.
- Trans fats.
- Hydrogenated fats.
- Too much alcohol.

TRANS FATS

The saturated animal fat we try so hard to avoid has in fact been replaced in our diet by the even more risky trans fats. These are the worst kind of fats, made by complex processing of natural oils at tremendously high temperatures to prolong shelf life; the living ingredients are killed to prevent the oil from turning rancid. They are known as *trans* fatty acids because they allow toxic substances to pass *through* the cell membranes. The human body had never encountered such unnatural fats as these before food processing came in. They are an obvious cancer risk.

WHERE DO I FIND TRANS FATS?

Margarines
Ordinary supermarket cooking oils
Pastry, cakes, biscuits, chocolate
Potato crisps and deep-fried snacks

**The fat they contain is usually labelled
'polyunsaturated fat'**

HYDROGENATED FAT

This fat is made by pumping hydrogen into vegetable oil at enormous pressure to solidify it, in order to make margarine—this is why butter is safer. We are naturally designed to take limited amounts of saturated animal fat. Unhydrogenated margarines are sold in health food shops and are now being introduced into supermarkets.

Fry with olive oil or butter

Avoid frying with nut, seed or soya oils because when polyunsaturated fat is damaged by heat it becomes toxic and creates rogue molecules called free radicals which damage healthy cells throughout the body.

WHERE DO I FIND ESSENTIAL FATS AND OILS?

Avocado pears
Fresh nuts in shells
Sunflower, pumpkin and sesame seeds
Fresh vegetables and green salad

Fresh oily fish:
Herrings, mackerel
Sardines, pilchards
Salmon, tuna, trout

Unrefined cold-pressed oils
(from health food shops)

Fresh wholefoods are the best sources of essential fats because the oils they contain are fresh and unprocessed.

MAKING UP THE DEFICIENCY

Extra virgin olive oil
(monounsaturated fat)
one to two tablespoonfuls per day

Unrefined safflower oil or sunflower oil
(polyunsaturated fat)
one dessertspoonful per day

Many of us have become so deficient over the years that we could never get enough essential oils to make up the deficiency from food alone.

How do I take the oil?

- It can be mixed into butter and other spreads to make them more spreadable. It softens the bread if it is dry and it keeps sandwiches moist.

- Dip your bread in it as Mediterranean people do.
- Blend it into soups or porridge before serving.
- Add it to rice before serving for a fresh, fruity taste.
- Make mayonnaise or French dressings with it.
- Add it to fruit juice or water and shake it up in a small screw-top jar. This takes the oily texture right away and you can then drink it or pour it over salad.

Cold-pressed oils are an acquired taste but you will soon learn to enjoy them. Safflower oil is more bland than sunflower oil and higher in polyunsaturates, too.

Polyunsaturated nut and seed oils need to be kept refrigerated once they have been opened. Protect them from light, because light is destructive to all the oils.

Extra virgin olive oil is very easy to fry with. It can be stored at room temperature.

Evening primrose oil can be taken (in capsules) instead of safflower or sunflower oil. It is mentally calming and a powerful tonic. It can be taken alone or combined with fish oil.

Linseeds or Linusit Gold (crushed linseeds sealed in foil packets) can be added to breakfast cereal. They are crushed to ease absorption and sealed to prevent deterioration of the oil.

Linseed oil (food grade) otherwise known as flax seed oil: 2–4 teaspoonfuls a day can be taken instead of fish oil.

It is perhaps less well known that, like evening primrose oil, this can have potent and far-reaching health benefits (it put bounce into my hair for the first time ever). The bottled oil works out much cheaper and is more effective than the capsules. It is supplied by food supplement companies: see Useful Addresses.

Blood test for levels of the various essential fatty acids
See Biolab under Useful Addresses.

CHECK YOUR DIET

Total daily calories average 1,800–2,200

FLUID
One litre at least

CONCENTRATED PROTEIN
2–4 ounces per day

CONCENTRATED STARCH
Up to about five helpings

FRESH FRUIT
5 pieces (about 500 g or one pound)

SALAD AND RAW VEGETABLES
At least 250 g (8 oz)

ESSENTIAL OILS
Extra virgin olive oil: 1–2 tablespoonfuls
Unrefined safflower or sunflower oil: 1 dessertspoonful

Keep animal fats to a minimum
including dairy products, especially cheese and cream

This is just a guide for the day.
Individual needs vary.

CHAPTER 9

Make Up Your Own Meals

When you first start following the Hay diet you may prefer to depend on the menus and meal lists given in Chapter 12. Sooner or later, however, you will want to make up the meals yourself, and this chapter is your guide. Don't worry too much initially about getting the food combinations right in every respect, just be guided by the circular food combining diagrams.

There is also a coded food index near the end of this chapter. You can look up any natural food to see whether it goes with an alkaline, starch or protein meal. Use the chart at the very end of the chapter to plan your meals for the week.

If you are staying with family or friends, why not buy them a food combining recipe book?

EVERY DAY

at least

one
alkaline
meal

one
starch
meal

one
protein
meal

Snack on neutral foods

NEVER MISS MEALS

NEUTRAL FOODS

These go with both starch meals and protein meals.
They can also be taken as a snack between meals:
VEGETABLES cooked and raw
except potatoes
SALADS
FATS AND OILS
including butter, cream and cream cheese
HERBS AND SPICES

*   *   *

RAISINS
NUTS AND SEEDS
Raisins are high in natural sugar.
Nuts average 10–25 per cent protein.
Sunflower and pumpkin seeds are also 25 per cent
protein, *so take them all in small quantities only*.

**With the exception of fats and oils, these foods are also
alkali-forming.**

PROTEIN-BASED
MEALS

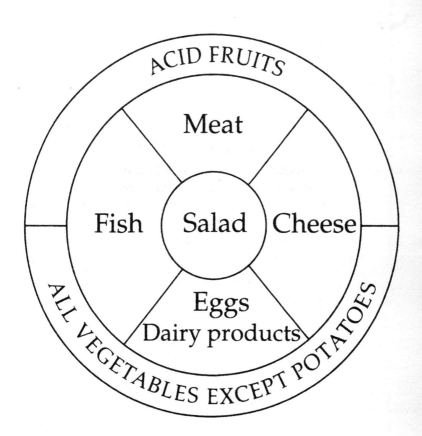

PROTEIN-BASED MEALS

Remember
Only CONCENTRATED protein foods
are kept entirely to separate protein-based meals:
MEAT, FISH, EGGS AND CHEESE

*   *   *

All vegetables are allowed except potatoes.
If you miss the potatoes,
serve extra vegetables instead.

Don't forget: no bread, pasta, rice or any other grains.

Protein meals are easy to prepare. The meat is served as usual, but without the potatoes. You will enjoy them, as they are so much lighter and more refreshing. There is no need to feel sluggish and sleepy after a meal like this: you can soon be ready for action again.

For better digestion:
- Only one kind of protein at a meal.
- Eat plenty of salad with concentrated protein.

And remember: we store very little protein, so never miss a protein meal—we must have one every day.

WHAT IS CONCENTRATED PROTEIN?

It is *animal* protein.
Concentrated protein foods are 20 per cent protein or more. They also contain fat, water and other nutrients.

- Vegetables, grains, milk and yoghurt also contain protein but always in smaller amounts.

- Dried beans, peas and lentils are not concentrated protein foods. Pulses go mainly with starch meals but there is nothing to stop you taking them with a protein meal too.

Which foods go with a protein meal?

Fish
Cheese
Acid fruits
Meat
Eggs

Acid fruits go with protein-based meals

They are not protein foods: they just require acid digestion like protein.

ACID FRUITS MEANS ALL FRUITS EXCEPT THOSE ON THE STARCH LIST.

Dried ACID fruits only with a protein meal: apricots, apple, peach, pineapple.

Melon is best eaten alone. It does not digest well with other foods.

Acid fruits eaten with starch foods are a common cause of bloating and wind.

Dairy products go with protein-based meals

- Hard cheese.
- All the softer crumbly cheeses.
- Soft, wet cheeses like cottage cheese.

Use hard cheeses in strict moderation only. Avoid processed cheese.

ONLY THE CHEESES MENTIONED ABOVE ARE CONCENTRATED PROTEIN.

The other dairy products are much less concentrated, but they still go with protein-based meals because they do not digest well with starch. They are:

Milk
Yoghurt
Fromage frais

Remember that butter, cream and cream cheese are neutral— they are mostly fat.

Keep dairy fats to a minimum

If you use strong cheese you need less of it. A light grating adds plenty of flavour.

● Fromage frais is only 7 per cent protein and very low in fat. Fat levels vary from 1 per cent to 8 per cent so it is a healthy substitute for cream.

Remember that milk does not digest well with meat, but you could use a little cream instead.

STARCH-BASED MEALS

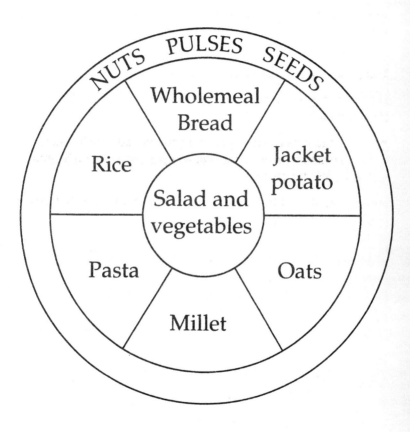

STARCH-BASED MEALS

Vegetarian meals with a difference

No hard cheese, no soft cheese, no yoghurt, no milk.
Only egg yolk is allowed.

*   *   *

ANY VEGETABLES
SALAD OF ALL KINDS
ANY NUTS AND SEEDS

*   *   *

POTATOES AND GRAINS
including millet,
wholemeal bread, wholewheat pasta, brown rice,
all the other grains.

*   *   *

BUTTER, CREAM AND NATURAL
CREAM CHEESE
are allowed
because they contain hardly any protein.

Remember that only CONCENTRATED starches are confined to separate starch-based meals:

- Concentrated starches are 20 per cent starch or more. Other vegetables do contain starch but always in smaller amounts.
- All the grains except millet are acid-forming.

Meals like this can be quite a challenge at first, but you will soon learn to make them rich and satisfying. In Chapter 12 there are plenty of meal suggestions and menus to get you started.

Only the sweetest fruits go with starch-based meals

This is because they are high in natural sugar, although they are not concentrated starch foods. Sugar and starch are both carbohydrate foods as starch turns to sugar in the body.

- Dates, figs and very sweet grapes are up to 50 per cent sugar.
- A very ripe banana may contain the equivalent of up to three teaspoonfuls of natural sugar.
- Although there is sugar in carrots, onions and parsnips, it is much less concentrated so they go with any meal.
- A little honey or maple syrup can be used very occasionally as a compromise.
- No artificial sweeteners—they are chemical additives.

In days gone by sugar was expensive and used only as a spice. Learn to sweeten foods naturally—see page 112.

Sugar and sweetened foods are not recommended, but if you want them for the occasional treat, remember that they go with starch meals.

Vegetable proteins go with starch-based meals

This is because they are not *concentrated* protein.

Why put pulses with starch meals?
Traditional dishes in many cultures combine grains with pulses, and of course vegetarians and vegans rely on this combination for much of their protein. Dr Hay also put the pulses with starch meals. Some people find them indigestible, but even if you do not, take them in moderation only, remembering that they are more acid-forming than grains.

DRIED PULSES
Peas, beans and lentils: these are mostly starch with only 5 per cent protein when cooked.
To make a complete protein: five tablespoons whole grain to one

tablespoon pulses. Home-cooked dried pulses are far more nutritious than canned ones.

Whole grains with beans or peas are a good combination. They are very sustaining and they help to stabilise blood sugar levels.

- Tinned baked beans combine with wholemeal toast to make a complete protein, but they are a compromise of course.
- Remember that sprouted pulses such as beanshoots are alkali-forming and very much easier to digest. They can be combined with any meal.

Enriching starch meals

Animal protein foods, including dairy products, are all complete proteins because they contain a full set of 22 amino acids, which are the individual components of protein, ready to be built into the body.

Vegetable proteins are incomplete
- Eight of the 22 amino acids cannot be manufactured in our own body and some of the eight are always missing from vegetable proteins.
- One food can be combined with another to complete the set, so that amino acids that are missing from one food will be present in the other. A small amount of complete protein will also enhance any vegetable protein.

Meals combined in this way are much more satisfying and more easily digested than animal proteins. Sustaining combinations of grains with beans, for example, are particularly important if you suffer from low blood sugar. But don't worry if you cannot always get the combinations right: experts believe that we have a small pool of amino acids which can be used to complete vegetable proteins when necessary.

The reason why natural, unprocessed vegetable proteins are actually easier to digest is because, unlike animal products such as cheese and meat, they are part of a whole and balanced food. We need a very varied diet to ensure that we get a wide enough selection of amino acids to meet all our needs.

Soya goes with starch meals

Soya is the only complete vegetable protein. It is taken with starch meals because it is not a concentrated protein.

Healthy soya products
Soya milk, soya beans, tofu.

- Soya milk is 4 per cent protein. Make sure it is marked 'unsweetened'. It is not a high calcium drink like cow's milk.
- Cooked soya beans are about 10 per cent protein. They need a strong-flavoured sauce to make them palatable.
- Tinned soya beans are available from health food shops and some supermarkets.
- TVP (textured vegetable protein) is highly processed and not recommended.

Tofu (white soya cheese)
Tofu is an important part of vegan diets and is especially popular in the Orient. It comes in firm white cakes or as 'silken' tofu, which is soft and creamy. It tastes nothing like dairy cheese, being very bland, but it does take up flavours from other foods very well. It is very versatile and highly nutritious:

- It contains 7–10 per cent protein.
- It is rich in calcium.

Tofu makes both sweet and savoury dishes. There are tempting recipes for tofu in *Food Combining for Vegetarians* by Jackie LeTissier.

STARCH MEALS:
TO MAKE A COMPLETE PROTEIN

Combine the food at the top of each section with one or more of the other foods.

RICE + Beans, peas, lentils Nuts Salad, raw vegetables	OATS + Soya milk Nuts, seeds
WHOLEMEAL BREAD + Nut butter and tahini Beans Tofu Lentil soup Pea soup	MILLET + Beans, peas, lentils Nuts, seeds Raw vegetables Salad Soya milk, tofu
RAW VEGETABLES AND SALAD + Rice, millet Mushrooms Brazil nuts Sesame seeds, tahini	POTATO + Soya milk SWEETCORN + Beans
PEANUTS + Any other nuts Sunflower seeds Pumpkin seeds	WHOLE WHEAT CEREALS + Soya milk Nuts, seeds

Soya milk instead of cow's milk with starch meals
Some people find that their digestion improves greatly when they stop taking cow's milk with their cereals. It can ferment with starch, causing indigestion or bloating and wind.

- If you cannot adapt to soya milk and you are unaffected by taking cow's milk with cereal, you can compromise.
- Remember that soya milk and tofu are processed foods, so take them in limited amounts only. They do not suit everybody.
- Rice 'milk' is another option.

Soya products are available from health food shops and larger supermarkets.

ALKALINE MEALS

Alkaline salad meals

Raw vegetables and salad form the basis of these meals.
Combine them with any of the following foods:

Natural yoghurt.
All fruit, both fresh and dried.
Almonds, hazelnuts, brazil nuts and pine nuts only: the other nuts are acid-forming.
Sunflower and pumpkin seeds

NOTE
- Only raw, untreated milk is alkali-forming. Pasteurised milk is acid-forming.
- Vegetable soup can also be taken with this meal (without potato).
- Use only fresh or sprouted beans and peas.
- Dried pulses are acid-forming, whereas sprouted pulses become alkali-forming and very highly nutritious. They are a 'superfood'.

Alkaline starch meals

Base your meal on jacket potato or millet and serve it with any of the other alkali-forming foods, *except yoghurt.*

ALKALINE MEALS

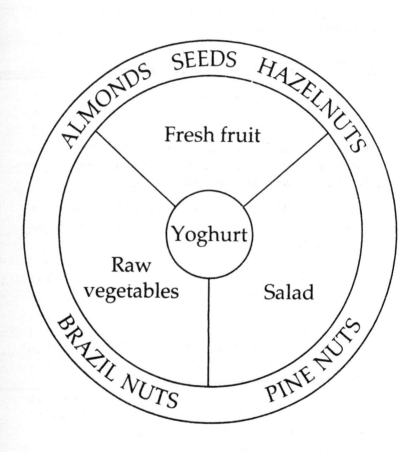

Cooked vegetables and *vegetable soup* are allowed.
The sweetest fruits only: bananas, yellow pears, grapes, dates and
   figs.

NOTE
You may need more than one starch meal a day to maintain
comfortable blood sugar levels.

Alkaline foods should make up the bulk of the Hay diet

An alkaline meal helps to ensure that we get enough alkali-
forming food over the day. If you cannot always fit one in, be sure
to balance each meal with plenty of fresh fruit and salad.
Remember that the more alkali-forming the diet is, the faster
and better the result. A balanced diet is essential, however, so
resist the temptation to eat only alkaline foods.

- Fats and oils are neutral but can be taken with alkaline meals.
- Fresh fruit or salad before a cooked meal helps digestion and
  reduces allergic reactions.
- Nuts and seeds can be easier to digest with fruit or salad. If
  they are soaked in water overnight in the refrigerator they
  become deliciously crisp, plump and tender.

Alkaline starches
- Jacket potatoes are alkali-forming only if you eat the skin,
  because the alkali-forming minerals lie just underneath it.
  Peeled potatoes are acid-forming.
- Millet is the only alkali-forming grain. It is therefore an
  important part of the Hay diet, and a filling way to maintain
  your alkaline balance. All the food combining books have
  recipes for millet. It is easy to prepare.
- Millet flakes can be used to make porridge and muesli. They
  are small, light flakes, similar to porridge oats. They are
  available from health food shops.

ALKALINE STARCH MEALS

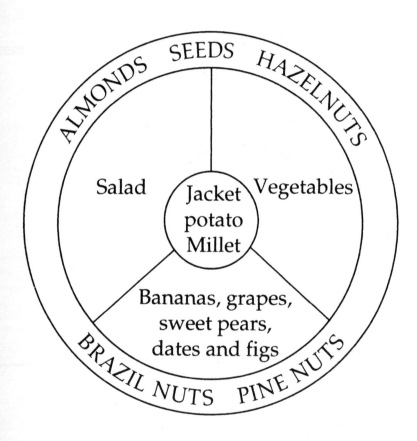

ALMONDS SEEDS HAZELNUTS

Salad   Jacket potato Millet   Vegetables

Bananas, grapes, sweet pears, dates and figs

BRAZIL NUTS   PINE NUTS

STEPS TO A NEW LIFE

1 Don't mix foods that fight!

Separate concentrated starches from concentrated protein.
Combine acid fruits with protein-based meals.
Combine very sweet fruits and sugar with starch-based meals.

2 Cut out all processed food

Replace it with natural wholefoods.
Gradually cut out sugar and all sweetened foods.
Learn to sweeten foods naturally.
Avoid food additives as far as possible.

3 Fresh fruit, salads and raw vegetables

These should eventually make up at least 50 per cent of the diet.

4 Change to more natural drinks

Reduce caffeine and alcohol if you take them to excess.

THE HAY DIET FOOD COMBINING CHART		
Do not mix starch with protein		
—combine—		—combine—
STARCH MEALS	NEUTRAL FOODS	PROTEIN MEALS
Potatoes	Vegetables *except potatoes*	Meat and fish
*		*
All grains: bread, rice, pasta	* Salads and herbs	Whole eggs
*	*	*
Dried beans, peas and lentils	Nuts and seeds	Hard cheese Soft cheeses
*	*	*
Soya milk, tofu	Fats and oils: butter and cream	All fruits *except those on the starch list*
*		
Egg yolk		
*		
Bananas Sweet pears Grapes Dates and figs		
*		
Honey *in small amounts*		

MAKE UP YOUR OWN MEALS

CHANGING COMBINATIONS

OUT	IN
Cheese sandwiches	Banana sandwiches
Meat sandwiches	Salad sandwiches
Fruit pie	Stewed fruit
Meat pie	Vegetable pie
Roast meat and roast potatoes	Meat with roast parsnips
Meat and potato pie	Vegetarian potato pie
Pasta with meat or cheese	Pasta with vegetarian sauce
Meat with rice	Vegetables with rice
Macaroni cheese	Cauliflower cheese
Cheese and biscuits	Apple and cheese
Egg on toast	Egg with grated cheese
Fish and chips	Fish with salad
Beefburger in a roll	Vegeburger in a roll

DRINKS—WHICH MEAL?

DRINK	STARCH	PROTEIN	ALKALINE
Tea	●	●	
Coffee	●	●	
Herb teas	●	●	●
Soya milk	●		
Fruit juices		●	●
Vegetable juices	●	●	●
Spring water	●	●	●
Milk is best taken as a snack between meals or with fruit for breakfast.			

MAKE UP YOUR OWN MEALS

ALCOHOL—WHICH MEAL?

ALCOHOL	STARCH	PROTEIN
Sweet wines	●	
Beer, lager	●	
Sweet liqueurs	●	
Dry cider		●
Dry wines		●
Spirits	●	●
Sweet wines and sweet liqueurs can cause blood sugar swings.		

EVERYDAY FOODS
Starch-based or Protein-based Meal?

S = Starch   P = Protein   N = Neutral
+ = Alkali-forming   − = Acid-forming

Almonds	N	+	Cherries	P	+
Apples	P	+	Chestnuts	S	−
Apricots	P	+	Chicken	P	−
Artichoke	N	+	Chickpeas	S	−
Asparagus	N	+	Chicory	N	+
Aubergine	N	+	Chinese leaves	N	+
Avocado pear	N	+	Clementines	P	+
Bamboo shoots	N	+	Cockles	P	−
Bananas	S	+	Coconut	N	−
Barley	S	−	Cod	P	−
Beans			Cornmeal (maize)	S	−
dried	S	−	Courgettes (zucchini)	N	+
fresh	N	+	Crab	P	−
Beanshoots	N	+	Cream	N	N
Beef	P	−	Cress	N	+
Beetroot	N	+	Cucumber	N	+
Blackberries	P	+	Dates	S	+
Blackcurrants	P	+	Duck	P	−
Bran	N	−	Eggs, whole	P	−
Brazil nuts	N	+	yolk only	N	−
Bread	S	−	Endive	N	+
Broad beans	N	+	Figs	S	+
Broccoli	N	+	Fish	P	−
Cabbage	N	+	Garlic	N	+
Carrots	N	+	Gooseberries	P	+
Cashew nuts	N	−	Grapefruit	P	+
Cauliflower	N	+	Grapes		
Celeriac	N	+	extra sweet	S	+
Celery	N	+	sharper taste	P	+
Cheese			Hazelnuts	N	+
cottage-type	P	−	Kale	N	+
cream cheese	N	N	Kohlrabi	N	+
crumbly cheese	P	−	Kiwi fruit	P	+
hard cheese	P	−	Leeks	N	+

Lemon	P	+	Plums	P	−
Lentils	S	−	Pomegranate	P	+
Lettuce	N	+	Potato		
Limes	P	+	jacket	S	+
Linseeds	N	+	peeled	S	−
Loganberries	P	+	Prunes	P	−
Lychees	P	+	Pumpkin seeds	N	+
Mango	P	+	Quinoa grain	S	−
Marrow	N	+	Radishes	N	+
Millet	S	+	Raisins	N	+
Mushrooms	N	+	Raspberries	P	+
Nectarine	P	+	Rhubarb	P	−
Oats	S	−	Rice, brown	S	−
oat bran	N	−	Runner beans	N	+
Okra	N	+	Rye	S	−
Olives	N	+	Satsumas	P	+
Onions	N	+	Sesame seeds	N	+
Oranges	P	+	Spinach	N	+
Papaya	P	+	Sprouted beans	N	+
Parsnips	N	+	Sprouted seeds	N	+
Passion fruit	P	+	Strawberries	P	+
Peaches	P	+	Sultanas	N	+
Peanuts (pulses)	S	−	Sunflower seeds	N	+
Pears			Swede	N	+
green	P	+	Sweetcorn	N	+
soft yellow	S	+	Sweet potato	S	+
Peas			Tofu	S	−
fresh	N	+	Tomatoes		
dried	S	−	fresh	N	+
Pecan nuts	N	−	cooked, tinned	P	−
Peppers	N	+	Turnip	N	+
Pine nuts	N	+	Walnuts	N	−
Pineapple	P	+	Watercress	N	+
Pistachios	N	−	Yams	S	+
Plantain	S	+	Yoghurt, natural	P	+

THE HAY DIET MADE EASY

HAY DIET MENU PLAN			
DAY	BREAKFAST	MIDDAY	EVENING
Mon			
Tues			
Wed			
Thurs			
Fri			
Sat			
Sun			

CHAPTER 10

Changing Over to Natural Food

An all-natural diet does mean spending more time in the kitchen, but if you persevere, and if you are reasonably fit, by the end of the first month you could be waking up so much earlier, and could be so much more clear-headed and energetic, that the extra preparation will no longer be a problem because you will have so much more time. If you are not well, each new change you make will give you the strength to make another.

A GUIDE TO PROCESSED FOODS

Bacon, ham, ham on the bone: all these are made from pork which has usually been chemically treated to make it pink.

Corned beef contains preservatives and is heavily salted.

Cornflakes: highly processed and often contain a surprising amount of sugar.

Diet yoghurts contain artificial sweeteners.

Dried soups and sauces: heavily salted and devitalised by heavy processing.

Frozen foods: some vitamins are destroyed when they are blanched; storage and cooking reduce them further. Nevertheless they are a valuable part of our diet.

Fruit yoghurts usually contain added sugar.

Gravy powder: very salty and often contains caramel colouring which is chemically produced.

Heavily spiced foods are very acid-forming.

Mayonnaise and other salad dressings: the oil they contain is usually highly processed, so make your own salad dressings with cold-pressed oil if you can.

Pickled foods are very acid and very salty.

Sausages usually contain colour and preservatives.

Stock cubes are very salty and often contain monosodium glutamate which can cause reactions.

Supermarket cold meats usually contain additives and salt. Look carefully at the small print on the labels.

Tinned meat of all kinds often contains a lot of salt. Look out for additives.

Tinned soups are also salty and they often contain monosodium glutamate which is a flavour enhancer. Look out for it in soups where the label quite correctly states that it contains no artificial colours or preservatives.

Tinned tomatoes are acid-forming.

Tinned white rice and other milk puddings: they contain added sugar, the grains are refined, and milk and grains are an incompatible food combination.

Vinegar is very acid; lemon juice or lime juice are better.

White semolina: use wholemeal semolina.

Why does processed food keep fresh for so much longer?

Packaged and tinned foods and drinks, which keep fresh for an unnaturally long time at room temperature or in the fridge, do not deteriorate because they are so deficient in living ingredients and so full of preservatives.

COMMERCIAL DRINKS

Alcohol-free beers are often full of additives which can affect sensitive people.

Cola drinks contain caffeine, caramel colouring and phosphoric acid, besides being loaded with sugar.

Diet drinks: remember that artificial sweeteners are chemical additives.

Fruit squashes contain sugar and preservatives.

See *E For Additives* by Maurice Hanssen for more information.

CHANGING OVER TO NATURAL FOOD

CHANGE OVER TO NATURAL FOOD

OUT	IN
Sugar and sweetened foods: Biscuits, cake, ice-cream Chocolate, sweets Sweet fruit yoghurts Diet yoghurts	A little honey Fresh fruit Fresh dairy cream Natural yoghurts with fresh fruit
White rice White bread White flour White pasta White crispbreads	Natural brown rice Wholemeal bread only Wholemeal flour Wholemeal pasta Wholemeal crispbreads
Cornflakes Instant oat cereals Puffed rice or wheat Sugary breakfast cereals	Shredded wheat Natural porridge oats Sugar-free muesli Wholewheat cereals
All margarines All ordinary supermarket cooking oils	Butter only *For cooking:* Butter, dripping, olive oil
Pickles and sauces Dried soups Salted nuts Potato crisps Salted snacks	Herbs and spices Home-made soups Plain, fresh nuts Sunflower seeds Pumpkin seeds
Kippers, smoked fish	Fresh or frozen fish
Processed meats: Supermarket cold meats Pork pies Bacon and ham Corned beef Sausages and beef burgers	*Any fresh, home-cooked meat:* Sliced roast meat Chops Stewing steak Liver, kidney Poultry
Textured vegetable protein (TVP)	Soya beans Tofu (soft soya cheese)

CHANGE OVER TO MORE NATURAL DRINKS

OUT	IN
Tea	Herb teas
Coffee	Cereal coffee Chicory Dandelion coffee
Chocolate drinks, cocoa	Carob drinks
Packet soup drinks	Home-made soup drinks
Canned soft drinks Fruit squashes Diet squashes, cola	Pure fruit juice diluted with sparkling spring water
Lemonade Glucose drinks Alcohol-free lager	Freshly squeezed lemon juice Sparkling spring water with a slice of lemon
Remember that milk is best taken between meals, or with fruit for breakfast	
WATER IS THE BEST DRINK	

CHAPTER 11

Preparing Natural Food

Throughout this chapter the recipe ideas have been coded according to their category—alkaline, starch, protein or neutral. These are the codes:

A = Alkaline   S = Starch meal   P = Protein meal   N = Neutral

The fresher the better

Fresh foods prepared from natural ingredients deteriorate rapidly, but the faster they spoil the more living ingredients they contain and the more invigorating they will be.

Food is best eaten as soon as possible after it is harvested. Home-grown vegetables are a good idea; so are those available fresh from country markets and Women's Institute markets, or bought directly from farms and nurseries.

KEEP IT FRESH

Salad cress, beanshoots and other sprouted pulses are 'super-foods' because they are still growing.

Salad cress: stand it in a small plastic box on the window-sill and keep it watered.

Celery sticks can be kept standing in a little water, ready to eat at any time.

Lettuce: keep it in a sealed plastic bowl with a lid which lets some light in. Add a very little water. There is no need to keep it in the fridge.

Peppers, aubergines, courgettes and carrots: buy the harder ones; they are fresher. They all keep better if refrigerated in a sealed plastic box.

All vegetables keep longer in the refrigerator: you can buy refrigerators with an exceptionally large drawer at the bottom.

FRESH HERBS

Bay leaves give a rich savoury aroma. Throw them away after cooking.

Marjoram is sometimes called the 'salt and pepper' plant. It is prolific and easy to grow.

Sage and thyme will also add flavour to a salad.

Fresh rosemary has a very powerful flavour.

Mint can be taken with salads, including fruit salads.

Lemon balm is prolific and very easy to grow. Add it to salads including fruit salad.

Dill: if you can find fresh dill chop lots of it finely into rice just before it is served.

Tarragon is a hardy plant whose leaves are aniseed-flavoured.

Dandelion leaves are actually highly nutritious salad greens, rich in potassium.

Land cress (American cress) tastes like watercress. Again it is prolific and easy to grow from seed. It grows right through the winter.

Herb teas

Any of these may be added to herb teas for extra flavour:
    Two or three cloves.
    One head of star anise.
    A curl of cinnamon bark.
    A squeeze of fresh orange or lemon juice.

Lemon balm, mint or sage tea:
    Use a sprig of fresh leaves and pour boiling water on them.
    Leave it to stand until it is cool enough to drink, then strain it.

Hot lemon with ginger:
Cut off a thin slice of root ginger, then peel it and dice it finely. Add boiling water and leave it to infuse until it is cool enough to drink. Add a squeeze of lemon juice.

WHOLE SPICES

Their flavour is fresh and exciting by comparison with the commercial ground spices. Use them sparingly as they have strong flavours.

Cardamom pods have a powerful aromatic flavour. Use three or four whole pods and remove them after cooking. Alternatively remove the tiny black seeds from inside the pods.
Cloves go well with cooked apples, rhubarb or dried fruit.
Juniper berries have a powerful and very distinctive flavour.
Whole nutmeg tastes deliciously fruity when freshly grated.
Fennel seeds taste strongly of liquorice or aniseed. Add them to muesli or cook them with rice.
Star anise has a sweet aniseed flavour. Good with cooked fruits such as apples.
Fresh root ginger: Chop a thin slice and add it to salads or stir-fries. Blend it into soups, or cook it with fruit.
Cinnamon sticks are curls of cinnamon bark with a fresh, fruity flavour. Add about an inch when cooking fruit.
Allspice seeds taste like cloves and cinnamon.
Coriander seeds have a strong hint of lemon. Their flavour is more delicate than other spices so you need to use more seeds.
Dried red chillies are very hot indeed. Half a chilli adds warmth to soups and stews.
Black peppercorns are strong too, so use them sparingly.
Black mustard seeds are very much milder than peppercorns.
Cumin seeds: cook with rice or meat for a pleasantly mild curry flavour.

If you have trouble digesting foods prepared with commercial ground spices, you may actually be able to tolerate them whole.

Your own freshly ground spices can also be easier on the digestion.

SWEETEN AND FLAVOUR IT NATURALLY

Starch-based meals

Banana adds sweetness.
Fresh root ginger goes well with banana.
Orange or lemon rind can be finely grated into rice or millet.
Dried dates can be cooked gently in a little water to make them fruity and soft. You can then purée them to make a sweet sauce.
Raisins go with fruit salad or they can be cooked with grains.
Honey: use only a very little; honey is refined by the bees!

Protein-based meals

Fruit juice and fresh fruit purées.
Cooked dried apricots can also be puréed to make a sauce.
Raisins in moderation—they can be soaked overnight in fruit juice.

With a starch or a protein meal

Try fresh coconut, desiccated coconut, coconut cream.

There are plenty more ideas in *Food Combining for Vegetarians* by Jackie LeTissier.

FRESH FOODS IN YOUR RECIPES

Mixed salad   N

Chop all salad items and fill a one-pint casserole dish with a selection from:

Lettuce	Watercress	Spring onions
Cucumber	Sweet peppers	Tomatoes
Raw leek	Sprouted beans	Raw cauliflower

Celery	Fennel	Brussels sprouts
Salad cress	Raw carrots	Sweetcorn
Chicory	Beetroot	Fresh peas
Beanshoots	Radishes	Raw cabbage

Sprinkle liberally with water to keep the salad alive. Cover it and keep in the fridge ready to use over the day. Nuts and seeds can be added before serving.

Salads go with any meal.

Raw vegetable soup   N

Quick and easy to make and a very powerful healer, like vegetable juices. Use a food processor or a powerful blender with a strong stainless steel blade, especially if you are blending raw carrot or beetroot (slice it finely first).

1 Chop or slice any mixture of raw vegetables and salad— tomato, cucumber, sweet peppers—enough to fill a mug.
2 Add fresh fruit if you like: apple, kiwi fruit, orange, lemon juice.
3 Add half a mug of water.
4 Flavour with any fresh herbs: sage, lemon balm, thyme or garlic.
5 Add a teaspoonful per serving of any cold-pressed oil.
6 Blend everything together.
7 Avocado can also be added for a more creamy soup.

Raw soup is also a very refreshing tonic: I would never have believed how much it could help, and in how many ways. Taken two or three times a day, with a little powdered psyllium husk if necessary (see p. 123) it can also effectively help stubborn constipation.

Introducing avocado pears

Avocados deserve special mention. They are alkali-forming, being a rich source of potassium, and they can be eaten at any meal. It comes as a surprise to most people that they are definitely not fattening; in fact avocados are a 'superfood', rich in essential oils, high in protein and vitamins C and B6.

Buying avocados
- If you can press your thumb into them very slightly, they are ready to use. As they ripen they should become uniformly soft like an orange.
- If they are hard, and soft only in certain places, they will be bruised. Buy the harder ones to ripen at home and eat later in the week. Refrigerate them, as they do not keep well once they are soft.
- To ripen them more quickly, keep them in a warm place such as an airing cupboard.

Serving avocados
Eat them straight away. They deteriorate very quickly.

- Avocados make a good snack to take to work. Just cut one in half and eat it with a teaspoon.
- Cut the avocado in half lengthways and remove the large stone.
- Fill with prawns, soft cheese or any other appropriate filling, and serve with salad.
- To keep half an avocado, smear the cut surface with olive oil.

AVOCADO CREAM   N

Deliciously refreshing, especially if you refrigerate the avocado first; it blends with other flavours very well. The easiest way to prepare it is in a large mug, using a hand blender. It makes a surprisingly large amount of cream.

- Cut a small avocado in half and scoop out the inside with a teaspoon. Chop one half into several pieces and liquidise it to a cream with a little water. You can eat the cream as it is.

- *You could also blend it with:*
A piece of banana;	A + S
Banana, chopped yellow pepper and corn oil;	N
Yoghurt or soft fruits;	A + P
Red or yellow pepper and olive oil;	N
Egg yolk and banana;	S
A little safflower or sesame oil for a nutty flavour;	N
Unrefined corn oil for a taste like chocolate—really!	N

Avocado cream is very easy to digest. It can ease digestive discomfort after a meal. It is ideal for sick people, babies and young children.

Fresh fruit drinks

A fresh orange squeezed into a glass of milk does not curdle.	P
Soft fruit blended into milk or soya milk: peach, nectarine, apricots, or strawberries.	P
Yoghurt drinks made with any fresh fruit.	A + P
Banana blended into soya milk.	S

Fresh fruit sauce

Use any soft blendable fruit:
    raspberries, strawberries, peaches, apricots.   A + P
Blend them together with a little fruit juice if necessary. Serve the sauce over fresh fruit.

Fresh fruit jelly   P

Dissolve 4 level teaspoons gelatine in a little warm water by standing the container in hot water while you stir it in. Make it up to one pint with cold fruit juice. Add any fresh acid fruits and refrigerate.

Banana sauce S

Blend a banana with water or soya milk.

Banana cream S

Blend a banana together with:
   Cream or coconut cream; S
   Avocado pear; S
   An equal quantity of chopped sweet pepper; S
   Rice; S
   A little root ginger. S

Fresh tomato sauce N

Skin the tomatoes and blend together. Add garlic, olive oil and fresh herbs to taste.

To skin a tomato:
- Score the skin lightly.
- Immerse it in boiling water for a minute or two until the skin loosens.
- Plunge it into cold water, then remove the skin.

Ripe tomatoes are easier to skin. You can also skin ripe peaches this way.

Cheese sauce (a compromise with protein meals) P

You could use potato flour to thicken the sauce as it has very little flavour of its own. If you use a strong-flavoured cheese you need less of it.

Red and yellow peppers N

Cut off large chunks to eat raw as a snack. They can taste deliciously sweet if you never have sugar.

Natural salad dressings

- Natural yoghurt with mint, chives or parsley.   A + P
- Avocado blended with raw garlic or herbs for a
  salad dip or dressing.   N
- French dressing made with olive oil and lemon or
  lime juice to taste.   A + P
- A little safflower or sesame oil added to salad before serving
  adds a nutty flavour. Use the light-coloured sesame oil; the
  darker one has a bitter flavour.

Home-made mayonnaise and French dressing: not with starch
meals because they contain lemon juice. *The Food Combining
Cookbook* by Erwina Lidolt contains a mayonnaise for starch
meals.

Frozen peas and sweetcorn with salad   N

To add them to a salad, just cover them with boiling water for
about a minute until they are defrosted. There is no need to cook
them.

Beetroots   N

They cook very quickly and easily in a microwave oven. Scrub
one and cook it in a small covered basin with about two tablespoonfuls of water. They take a little longer to cook than a jacket
potato, and can also be served hot.

Home-made vegetable soups   S

Use a cheap hand blender to blend the vegetables in the saucepan. Cook potato on its own or with other vegetables:
   Leek, carrot, swede, parsnip, onion.

When cooked:
1 Set aside some of the cooked vegetables to add to the soup
   after blending.

2 Flavour it by adding fresh garlic, root ginger or fresh herbs.
3 Add 1 teaspoon extra virgin olive oil per serving.
4 Blend the potato and other ingredients together.
5 Add the pieces of cooked vegetables which you set aside.
6 Cooked beans, peas, sweetcorn, or mushrooms can also be added afterwards.

Individual portions can be frozen.

Variations
1 Equal quantities of potato, carrot and onion.
2 Two parts potato to one part each carrot and parsnip.

Quick potato soup S

A thicker soup with a better flavour.
    Microwave a jacket potato. Cover it with cold water for a minute or two to loosen the skin, then remove it. Chop it roughly, cover it with water and prepare it as for the previous recipe.

Variations
Raw chopped green pepper blended into it makes it the colour of avocado cream.
Blend it with cooked butter beans.
It makes a creamy coating sauce over steamed vegetables.

Steamed vegetables N

Steaming vegetables leaves them with a much firmer texture and twice the flavour. Steamed potatoes have a very appetising sheen and they do not break up as they may when boiled.

Yams S

Yams are large root vegetables, sometimes weighing several pounds. Chopped, boiled yam blended with oil makes a deliciously thick and creamy soup, much thicker and more filling than potato soup. You can buy yams from ethnic shops and from enterprising greengrocers. Make sure they are fresh and very white inside, and refrigerate them as they do not keep fresh for long.

Cooking dried beans S

- Boil dried beans rapidly for ten minutes, then simmer until they are cooked. Unless they are boiled first they may cause digestive problems.
- Do not add salt to dried beans or peas while cooking because it prevents them from going soft and they will remain hard however long you cook them!
- When cooked they can be open frozen on trays and kept ready for when you need them.
- Tins of beans without sugar or salt can be found in health food shops.

Brown rice S

It has a good nutty flavour and the grains are less inclined to stick together than those of refined rice. It takes about forty minutes to cook in the usual way.

Variations
Cook it with any of these:
    Finely chopped carrot and brown lentils and a bay leaf.
    Black-eye beans.
    Cumin seeds, white mustard seeds or fennel seeds.

The most delicious brown rice comes from health food shops or market stalls. The brown rice bought in machine-sealed plastic packets from supermarkets often tastes quite unpleasant; the difference is quite remarkable.

Creamy brown rice porridge S

A slow cooker makes the softest rice. Brown rice boiled in the ordinary way can be gritty when blended.

Cooking method:
1 7 heaped tablespoonfuls rice to 2 pints water.
2 Rinse the rice with boiling water and strain it.
3 Pour boiling water onto it.

Flavouring:
Add half a teaspoonful of whole spice seeds:
    Fennel, allspice or juniper berries;
    or 1 teaspoon coriander seeds.

Leave it to cook for at least six hours in the slow cooker; if you cook it overnight you can wake up to fresh porridge.
    If you need the rice in a hurry you can finish cooking it by putting the crockpot in the microwave oven.

When cooked:
Use a hand blender and blend it in the crockpot. Blend the rice with one teaspoonful of extra virgin olive oil per serving. The oil makes it light and creamy and turns it white like milk. Rice cooked this way is easier to digest and absorb.

Variations
Blend individual servings of rice with banana or creamed coconut.

Individual portions can be frozen: cool it quickly by placing the crockpot in a bowl of cold water.

NOTE
A slow cooker can often be bought very cheaply from a car boot sale, but have it checked by an electrician before you use it.

Quick rice flake porridge S

Brown rice flakes are available from health food shops.

Cooking method:
1   1 tablespoon brown rice flakes to half a pint of cold water.
2   It helps to soak the flakes for a few minutes before cooking.
3   Cook slowly until thick.
4   Cook it with raisins for extra sweetness.

Microwaved rice flakes
Use a deep bowl to stop it from boiling over. Heat on full power for two minutes, then simmer for ten minutes on defrost setting.

INTRODUCING THE OTHER GRAINS

The more varied the diet, the quicker the results.

Millet S

This is a staple food in parts of Africa and Asia. It can also be bought as millet flakes or millet flour. It is alkali-forming and gluten-free.

Boiled millet
Cook as for rice. It goes well with coriander seeds and lemon rind, sweetcorn and carrot.

CREAMED MILLET PUDDING S
A deliciously light, smooth pudding, similar to semolina, but without milk. It works best in a slow cooker using the same quantities and the same method as for rice porridge.

Pot barley S

This is the natural whole grain. It needs long, slow cooking— again a slow cooker is ideal. Soak the barley overnight for quicker cooking. You can also buy barley flour. Barley is lower in gluten than wheat.

- It is naturally sweet and goes well with coriander seeds. It makes a good soya milk pudding, a delicious change from rice.
- You can make porridge with it following the recipe for brown rice porridge.
- It can also be cooked in a saucepan and used for savoury dishes instead of rice.
- It can be added to vegetable stews and casseroles.

Oat groats   S

This is the whole oat grain, as sweet and delicious as barley.

Buckwheat   S

Buckwheat is not actually wheat at all, but is related to rhubarb. It is gluten-free and can be bought as whole grains, raw or roasted. Roasted buckwheat has a slightly bitter flavour; raw buckwheat is the natural grain and is a lighter colour. You can also buy buckwheat flour and pasta.

NOTE
Kasha is a buckwheat cereal dish popular in eastern Europe. It is cooked slowly and served with olive oil, sesame oil or butter. This, too, cooks well in a slow cooker.

Quinoa   S

This is a highly nutritious gluten-free grain, a tiny round seed used since ancient times in South America. It can be mixed with other grains or added to soups. Rinse it well in a fine sieve with boiling water before cooking, otherwise it can taste slightly bitter. It cooks in ten minutes. Quinoa is somewhat thin and watery when cooked and not really suitable for puddings.

Cornmeal (maize) S

This is used extensively in North and South America. In Europe it is used to make polenta. There are recipes for sweet and savoury polenta in *The Food Combining for Health Cookbook* by Jean Joice and Jackie LeTissier and for polenta custard in *Food Combining for Vegetarians* by Jackie LeTissier.

Powdered psyllium husks (pronounced 'silium') N

Psyllium is a plant grown in India where it has been used for thousands of years. The powder is a very useful thickener for cold dishes as it is practically tasteless and thickens almost instantly, without cooking.

Its chief use is as a bulking agent for bowel problems:
- In constipation it increases the bulk so that the bowel muscles can get a better grip on the food and move it through the gut more easily.
- It relieves diarrhoea by absorbing the water.
- It can also effectively reduce embarassing wind and rumbling in the gut.
- It is well tolerated by people who cannot take bran.

It contains no additives and can be bought loose in a drum. See Useful Addresses for supplier.

CHAPTER 12

Meals and Menus

Here are some simple ideas to enable you to select a meal or a day's meals quickly and easily. They will help you until you get more used to food combining. You do not necessarily have to know, when you begin, which foods are starch and which foods are protein: just select from the appropriate lists or consult the menus. You may find it easier to plan a week's meals and shop for them in advance.

In the following pages you will find lists of neutral foods, alkaline, starch and protein meals, and suggested menus for two weeks, as well as ideas for packed lunches. Just take your choice. If a suggested fruit or vegetable is out of season, choose a substitute from the coded list on page 102.

Remember

Every day you need at least one alkaline meal, one starch-based meal and one protein-based meal.

NEUTRAL FOOD

Salads that go with any meal

Sliced beetroot, peas, onion rings and watercress.
Cucumber, tomato and salad cress.
Sliced tomatoes with onion rings.
Chopped apple, celery and nuts or raisins.
Chopped onion, raw cauliflower and sunflower seeds.
Chopped fennel, raw cauliflower and pumpkin seeds.
Grated carrot, raisins and sweetcorn.
Chopped peppers, sweetcorn and tomato.

Sliced avocado pear with tomato and onion rings.
Sprouted beans and sweetcorn piled onto lettuce leaves.
Raw cabbage shredded with apple or onion.

You could also add chopped fresh herbs, cold-pressed oil and lemon juice.

Quick snacks

Avocado pear	Raw carrot
Tomatoes	Head of chicory
Celery sticks	Chunks of red or yellow pepper

LIGHT ALKALINE MEALS

Drinks

- Herbal tea.
- Fruit juice or spring water.
- A liquidised melon makes a refreshing drink.

Fruit breakfasts or desserts

Choose any fruits, with or without natural yoghurt.

Apple	Orange	Grapefruit
Pear	Pineapple	Kiwi fruit
Banana	Grapes	Mango
Nectarine	Peach	Strawberries
Blackberries	Raspberries	Melon

Nutty snacks

- Almonds, hazelnuts, brazils or pine nuts.
- Sunflower seeds or pumpkin seeds.
- Nuts and raisins.
- Banana or a raw carrot with a handful of nuts or seeds.

ALKALINE SALAD MEALS

Fresh fruit, with or without natural yoghurt.
Salad of all kinds, with:
   almonds, hazelnuts, brazil nuts, or pine nuts.
Served plain, with French dressing or a yoghurt-based dressing.

You may also have:
   Vegetable soup without potato.
   Sprouted pulses only.

NOTE
No dried beans or peas.

ALKALINE STARCH MEALS

Drinks

- Herbal teas.
- Grape juice or spring water.
- Vegetable juice.

Fruit and nut breakfasts

- Banana, grapes, sweet pear.
- Banana, dates or figs with:
   almonds, hazelnuts, brazil nuts, pine nuts.
- Sunflower or pumpkin seeds.

Millet breakfasts

- Muesli: millet flakes with raisins, sunflower seeds, sliced banana.
- Millet porridge: millet flakes cooked with dates or raisins.
- Banana blended with millet.

Lunches

- Vegetable soup (no pulses).
- *Jacket potato and:*
    vegetarian sauce.
    light tahini.
    vegetable casserole.
    ratatouille.
- *Served with salad and:*
    almonds, hazelnuts, or pine nuts.
    sunflower seeds or pumpkin seeds.
- *Spiced millet mixed with:*
    sweetcorn, raisins and grated lemon rind.
    chopped celery, tomato and raw onion, pine nuts.
- Corn on the cob with salad.

DESSERTS
   Banana, sweet pear, grapes, dates, figs.
   Spiced millet with banana, dates and orange rind.
   Millet blended with banana.
   Creamed millet pudding with pears.
No yoghurt or milk.

ORDINARY STARCH MEALS

Vegetarian sandwiches only

Use butter, not margarine in your sandwiches.

Savoury sandwich fillings

Nut butter and cucumber or tomato	Beetroot, onion rings, watercress
Sliced tomato with onion rings	Sliced jacket potato with yeast extract
Cream cheese, yeast extract, salad cress	Vegetable paté with tomato
Yeast extract with egg yolk	Lettuce and yeast extract
	Light tahini with cucumber

Hummus   Sliced or mashed avocado
Mustard and lettuce   pear (eat it straight away,
Sliced tofu with yeast extract   it soon turns brown)

Wholemeal crispbreads, crackers, rice cakes and oatcakes can all
be topped with sandwich fillings.

REMEMBER

No apple or orange with your sandwiches; no cheese, meat,
whole egg or fish.

Use only 100 per cent wholemeal bread—stoneground is best.
'Brown' and granary breads contain varying amounts of white
flour. Health food shops sell delicious nut butters, but avoid
peanut butter if possible. Tahini is a tasty sesame seed spread.
Light tahini is made from hulled seeds; dark tahini is prepared
from whole seeds and tastes slightly bitter.

Sweet sandwich fillings
   Banana and honey   Banana with nut butter
   Date and banana   Mashed banana with coconut
   Banana with cream or   Banana mashed with ground
      cream cheese   almonds

Open sandwiches
   Cream cheese,   Nut butter with sliced
      banana, walnuts   tomato, cucumber and
   Mashed banana,   onion
      dates, cream,   Any vegetable paté with nuts
      chopped nuts   and salad
   Hummus piled with   Mashed avocado and sliced
      salad   tomato with mixed salad

Toasted sandwiches filled with banana or beans.
Wholemeal pitta bread stuffed with beans, salad or banana.

STARCH-BASED MEALS

Drinks

- Weak tea or coffee.
- Spring water or grape juice.
- Soya milk.

Cereal breakfasts

- Shredded wheat.
- Wheatflakes.
- Fruit and fibre cereal.
- Wholewheat breakfast biscuits.
- Sugar-free muesli:
  Oatflakes with flaked almonds, sunflower seeds, pumpkin seeds or raisins.
- Porridge.

Serve cereals with soya milk or liquidised banana.

Breakfasts based on wholemeal toast

- Butter.
- Lightly cooked mushrooms or tomatoes.
- Mashed banana.
- Scrambled egg yolks.
- Hummus and walnuts.
- Mashed avocado with sliced tomatoes and onion rings.

Light starch lunches

These can all be accompanied by a salad.

Lentil soup	Bean and vegetable soup
Potato soup	Salad rolls or sandwiches
Beans on toast	Wholemeal spaghetti on toast
Vegeburger in a roll	Jacket potato

A jacket potato and . . .

Butter	Corn on the cob	Vegetable
Cream cheese	Vegetarian sauce	casserole
Hummus	Cold pressed oil	Mushrooms and
Vegetable stir-fry	Beans	onions
Light tahini	Ratatouille	

Served with mixed salad.

Main starch-based meals

Serve with:

- Any vegetables, including potatoes.
- Salad, pasta, rice or bread.

HOT LUNCHES

- Nut roast with vegetarian sauce.
- Vegetable stir-fry with:
  cashew nuts, sesame seeds or small cubes of tofu.
- Spicy bean and vegetable stew.
- New potato stew with beans, whole onions and root vegetables.
- Vegetarian cottage pie.
- Steamed root vegetable mixture with vegetarian sauce.
- Vegetable curry with chapatis and poppadoms.
- Potato and vegetable cakes made with egg yolk.

Wholewheat pasta
- Pasta shapes, mixed vegetables and vegetarian sauce.
- Spaghetti, vegetables, vegetarian sauce.
- Wholewheat chinese noodles (they cook in four minutes).

Brown rice with . . .
- Vegetable curry and curry sauce.
- Fresh chopped cucumber, peas, spring onions and mint.

- Sweetcorn, red pepper, pine nuts, grated lemon rind, olive oil.
- Fried rice with onions, mushrooms and peas.
- Stir-fried vegetables.
- Ratatouille (aubergines, peppers and tomatoes).
- Chopped carrot and lentils (cooked with spicy rice).
- Baked beans mixed with fried mushrooms and onions to make a sauce.
- Curried beans mixed with cooked vegetables to make a sauce.
- Chilli beans mixed with sweetcorn and chopped tomatoes to make a sauce.
- Cold mixed beans and salad.

Millet, pot barley, or buckwheat can be used instead of rice.

Desserts with starch-based meals

- Banana, grapes, yellow pear.
- Dates or figs, fresh or dried.
- Sliced banana with:
  dates and walnuts, whipped cream.
- *Nuts of any kind*, including fresh coconut.
- *Brown rice or any other grain with:*
  banana, raisins, pine nuts and grated orange or
      lemon rind.
  Blend rice with a banana or coconut cream.
- *Use soya milk for:*
  banana custard (sugar free);
  spiced milk puddings.
- *Rice pudding with:*
  raisins, sliced banana or pears.

For millet desserts see alkaline starch meals (p. 127).

Sweet biscuits, cakes, pastries and sweet desserts go with starch meals but strictly speaking are not recommended.

PROTEIN-BASED MEALS

Drinks

- Weak tea or coffee.
- Fruit juice or vegetable juice.
- Spring water.

Protein breakfasts

- Fromage frais with mixed fruits.
- Cottage cheese with walnuts.
- Cheese with apple, celery, pineapple or grapes.
- Eggs fried with mushrooms and tomatoes.
- Scrambled egg mixed with chopped onion and tomato.
- Poached eggs with grated cheese, sliced tomatoes and onion rings.
- Ripe tomatoes cut in half, topped with grated cheese and grilled.

Light protein lunches with mixed salad

Grated cheese	Boiled egg
Sliced meat	Chicken leg
Fish	Any soft white cheese

Main protein meals

Serve with salad or any cooked vegetables except potato.

No bread, rice or pasta.

MEAT DISHES
- Meat and vegetable soup without potato.
- Casseroles, stews.
- Roasts, grills.
- Grilled: chops, pork cutlets, lamb cutlets.
- Roast pork with apple sauce

- *Minced meat*
    in a stew with mixed vegetables.
    hotpot topped with sliced aubergines or parsnips.
    chilli con carne (spiced minced beef with red kidney beans).
- Beefburgers, no additives.
- Beef stroganoff.
- Meat stir-fries, with beanshoots.
- Liver or kidney fried with mushrooms, onions and tomatoes.
- Steak and kidney with mushrooms and root vegetables.
- Roast duck with orange sauce.
- Meat curry—serve over lightly cooked white cabbage instead of rice.

FISH
- Grilled fresh herring, sardines or mackerel.
- Oily fish baked with butter in foil.
- Cod roes.

White fish
- Baked or grilled with butter.
- With mayonnaise and salad.
- In cheese sauce.
- With cauliflower cheese.

Other fish
- Salmon, tuna.
- Pilchards, herring roes.
- Sardine and tomato salad with onion rings, coleslaw and salad.
- Salmon and cucumber salad.

Shellfish of all kinds
- Prawns, shrimps, crab, lobster.
- Avocado pear with prawns.
- Prawn cocktail—prawns with lettuce.

Protein-based vegetarian meals

- Grated cheese salad.
- Cubes of white cheese with crunchy salad.
- Egg salad.
- Curried eggs.
- Egg mayonnaise.
- *Omelettes*
  mushroom, cheese and sweetcorn, or tomato.
  Spanish omelette made with vegetables except potato.
- Scrambled egg and sweetcorn and chopped peppers.
- Soft cheese with sweetcorn, peppers and salad.
- Cottage cheese with a little strong grated cheddar cheese.
- Avocado pear filled with soft cheese.

Cheese sauce dishes
- Cauliflower cheese topped with sliced tomato.
- Mixed vegetables in cheese sauce.
- Whole leeks in cheese sauce.
- Poached eggs in cheese sauce.
- Hard-boiled eggs in cheese sauce.
- Poached eggs on a bed of broccoli or spinach, covered with cheese sauce.

Desserts with protein-based meals

- Any fresh, acid fruits.
- Hot spiced dried apricots with yoghurt.
- Fresh fruit jelly with cream.
- Egg custard with nutmeg.
- Baked apple with cream.
- Natural fromage frais with soft fruits.
- Cottage cheese mixed with any acid fruits.
- Natural yoghurt with chopped fresh fruit.
- *Yoghurt*
  blended with soft fruits.
  with chopped nuts.

- Prunes with citrus fruit.
- Fruit salad mixed with a few cubes of white cheese.
- Fresh fruit salad with dried apricots and prunes.
- Any cooked fruit with fresh fruit or dried fruit added: chopped orange, kiwi fruit, lemon juice.
- Cooked dried apricots with yoghurt.
- Stewed apple with raisins and cream.
- *Tinned fruit in natural juice* can be used as a base to which fresh fruit can be added.

EATING OUT

Light lunches—starch-based meals

Vegetable soup and a
   wholemeal roll
Baked beans on toast
Bread roll filled with salad

Salad sandwiches
Jacket potato and salad
Fresh fruit: Banana,
   grapes, sweet pear

Main starch meals

You would get the widest selection at a vegetarian or wholefood restaurant. Eastern cultures have a rich tradition of vegetarian cooking: there are many exciting Indian, Chinese and Middle Eastern rice dishes without meat.

Protein meals

Meat or fish with vegetables
   or salad
Omelette and salad

Cheese or egg salad
Fruit salad or fresh acid
   fruits

Protein meals are simple to select: just omit the potatoes, rice and pasta and don't have any bread. There is no need to worry about small amounts of starch in gravy and sauces.

Teatime—starch meals

Bread rolls filled with salad.
Banana, sweet pear, grapes.

An occasional sweet treat will be all right unless you are very unwell.

MENUS WEEK ONE A = Alkaline S = Starch P = Protein		
BREAKFAST	**LUNCH**	**EVENING MEAL**
Sliced apple Yoghurt with flaked almonds A	Banana toasted sandwich Grapes Hazelnuts and raisins S	Grilled cod and butter Carrots and peas, cauliflower Fresh orange P
Avocado pear and banana blended together with water A	Vegetable stir-fry with sesame seeds Jacket potato Yellow pear A	Lamb chop, mushrooms, tomatoes, broccoli, carrots Fruit salad: Pineapple and fresh orange P
Millet porridge with raisins A	Corn on the cob, grated carrot, sliced beetroot, onion rings, green salad Fresh coconut A	Grilled steak, mushrooms, tomato, cucumber, green salad Cooked apple with fresh kiwi fruit and single cream P
Banana split lengthways with whipped cream and chopped nuts A	Mixed salad Lentil soup, wholemeal roll Avocado blended with cream S	Poached eggs, grated cheese Sweetcorn, chopped peppers, carrots Fresh green pear P
Sliced apple, blackberries Greek yoghurt A	Savoury brown rice with mixed beans and sweetcorn Mixed salad Dates and walnuts S	Diced turkey stew Mixed vegetables Fresh fruit salad: Orange and kiwi fruit P
Sugar-free muesli, soya milk Sliced banana S	Jacket potato, sliced avocado Mixed beans and sweetcorn with chopped onion and peppers Green salad Nuts and raisins A	Beef casserole Mushrooms, tomatoes, carrots, brussels sprouts Fruit juice jelly with pineapple P
Large slice of melon A	Roast pork, apple sauce Roast parsnips, carrots, broccoli Sliced peaches and mixed soft fruits P	Whole rye crispbreads Nut butter Sliced tomato Avocado and banana cream with walnuts S

MENUS WEEK TWO
A = Alkaline   S = Starch   P = Protein

BREAKFAST	LUNCH	EVENING MEAL

Shredded wheat, raisins
Soya milk
 	
S
	Savoury millet,
	  sweetcorn, peppers,
	  pine nuts, salad
	Sweet pear
	
	A
		Chicken and mushroom
		  casserole
		Cabbage, carrots, runner
		  beans
		Fresh mango
		
		P

Chopped grapefruit and
  orange
Brazil nuts and raisins
 	
A
	Vegetable pie
	Stir-fried vegetables
	Cashew nuts, salad
	Sweet grapes
	
	S
		Sliced beetroot, onion
		  rings, watercress
		Cheese omelette
		Mushrooms, tomatoes,
		  peas, carrots
		Fresh orange
		
		P

Mashed banana on
  wholemeal toast
  topped with walnuts
 	
S
	Jacket potato, light tahini
	Sweetcorn and peppers
	Tomato, cucumber,
	  watercress
	Fresh figs
	
	A
		Liver and onions
		Carrots and swede
		  mashed together,
		  cabbage
		Fruit salad:
		  Pineapple and orange
		
		P

Nectarine with yoghurt
 	
A
	Vegetable soup
	Pitta bread and salad
	Yellow pear
	
	S
		Grilled plaice, grated
		  cheese
		Carrots and peas, kale
		Sliced apples and
		  peaches
		
		P

Hazelnuts blended with yoghurt, chopped pear A	Vegetable soup Nut roast with salad Fresh dates S	Minced lamb Carrots, peas, broccoli Raspberries and cream P

Open sandwich:
  Wholemeal bread, nut
butter
Sliced banana and dates
 	
S
	Large fruit salad:
	  Fresh and dried fruit
	Hazelnuts and sunflower
	  seeds
	
	A
		Cauliflower cheese
		Poached egg, sliced
		  tomato, sweetcorn,
		  carrots
		Chopped orange with
		  raisins
		
		P

Strawberries and natural
  yoghurt
 	
A
	Roast chicken, roast
	  parsnips
	Broccoli and carrots
	Sliced kiwi fruit and
	  orange
	
	P
		Hummus dip with raw
		  vegetable sticks
		Banana and honey
		  sandwiches
		Whipped cream and
		  chopped walnuts
		
		S

PACKED LUNCHES

PROTEIN	STARCH	ALKALINE
Chicken leg Sliced tomato and cucumber Fresh peach	Wholemeal roll filled with lettuce and tomato Lentil and vegetable soup	Savoury yoghurt dip with mint and cucumber Carrot and celery sticks Nectarine
Crunchy mixed salad with grated cheese and walnuts Green pear	Hummus dip Carrot, celery sticks Rye crispbreads with butter	Head of chicory Natural yoghurt with apricots and almonds
Hard-boiled egg Mayonnaise Mixed salad Kiwi fruit	Cold rice salad: Sweetcorn, beans, chopped leek Sweet grapes	Cold new potatoes in skins Mixed salad with sweetcorn Sunflower seeds
Cheese and pineapple Mixed salad Fresh apricots	Oatcakes and nut butter Crunchy mixed salad Mixed nuts	Large orange Natural yoghurt Brazil nuts and raisins
Avocado pear with fromage frais Hazelnuts and raisins	Pitta bread filled with mixed beans and salad Banana	Cold sliced jacket potato Cruncy salad with pumpkin seeds Dates and banana
Small tin of fish Sliced tomatoes, onion rings Crunchy salad, fresh orange	Vegeburger in a roll Crunchy salad with sunflower seeds	Raw carrots and celery Handful of hazelnuts Banana and raisins
Soft ricotta cheese Chopped apple and pineapple Fresh mango	Kidney beans and sweetcorn with sesame oil and crunchy mixed salad Crispbreads spread with yeast extract	Mixed soft fruits Natural yoghurt Brazil nuts
Slices of cold roast meat Mixed salad Fresh peach	Mixed salad Nut butter and tomato sandwiches Fresh coconut	Mixed salad, sprouted pulses Freshly sliced avocado pear Fresh strawberries

Introducing Complementary Medicine

Complementary medicine is actually the traditional art of medicine—it was all we had before drugs and technology came in. Nowadays it is combined with the best of modern scientific research and is mainly practised by the health practitioners. It consists of safe treatments which are powerful, yet gentle and humane; they have been found to work over centuries of human experience. They are based on ways of activating the body's natural healing mechanism and restoring its natural balance. This is a huge and exciting field of medicine; it deserves to be better known.

All types of complementary therapy work on the causes of illness; they treat the person as a whole and can be surprisingly powerful. Patient and practitioner work together to change the diet and lifestyle that led to the illness. These methods can be used alongside conventional medicine, although of course you must not give up any prescribed medicine until you have recovered enough to do without it; you should consult your doctor about this.

Genuine and powerful alternatives to drugs and sometimes even routine operations do exist in complementary medicine—there are safer, less expensive and more effective ways of dealing with most everyday problems. And while scientific proof is essential for newly developed medical treatments, natural methods are safe enough to use without it. The proof is in the results and they are very convincing.

Diet before drugs

The nutritional approach to illness is extremely reliable; it will help most people, provided they can keep strictly to their diet.

All types of therapy benefit from nutritional support. Increasing numbers of people are turning to self-help books such as this one in their search for drug-free solutions, and the fewer drugs you have taken in your life, the faster and more complete your recovery will be when you try natural methods.

Doctors are trained to look for evidence of actual disease or damage. If they do not find it they are not seriously concerned with the many minor ailments which lead up to it, often putting them down to stress. This is where complementary medicine comes into its own: it offers much constructive help and understanding, especially since many health practitioners have suffered themselves and found answers in their own particular therapy. They have had to redraw their map of reality in a slow and painful way, as I have myself. They know that the real cures come largely by our own efforts.

REDUCING DRUG DEPENDENCE

Be very careful about reducing any prescribed drugs, because unless you deal with the underlying causes of your illness first, the symptoms will return. Wait until you have considerably recovered your strength, and consult your doctor before making any changes in your dosage: it needs to be done very gradually indeed. Everybody accepts that drugs have their place and that they save many lives, but when they are taken long term for chronic conditions they do not halt the disease process, they merely control it by suppressing the symptoms. This approach only drives it deeper into the body and prolongs the illness.

This is what can happen if you have unrecognised nutritional problems:
- The drug helps at first, sometimes in a dramatic way.
- If serious attention is not paid to the diet, the underlying illness progresses under cover of the drug.
- As your health continues to deteriorate, new symptoms

appear, some of which will be unrecognised side-effects of the drug.

- Ever-increasing doses of the drug will be required to keep the symptoms under control.
- Attempts to reduce the drug usually fail because the symptoms come back.

Eventually the problems in the diet overpower the drug and it no longer helps. By this time many people have become so addicted that they are powerless to give it up. They are now very sick and in metabolic chaos. We all know of people who are hopelessly ill despite taking a variety of medicines. In this situation they are often referred for psychiatry.

WARNING: Long-term tranquillisers, antidepressants and steroids

If you are taking any powerful drugs long term it can be dangerous to cut them down too quickly, especially if you have not investigated your diet. Find a doctor who specialises in nutritional medicine and stay in close touch with your GP, too.

THIS IS THE DANGER

Taking the drugs away too soon could be like taking the lid off a boiling saucepan. The full extent of the underlying illness would be exposed, putting you in a desperate state, in crisis. Without its usual treatment the illness could rapidly run further out of control, resulting in a devastating shock to the system which could set you back a very long way. Many of us are so desperate to cut down on our drugs that this predicament is not uncommon. It happened to me.

WARNING: The sudden withdrawal of steroid drugs can be life-threatening.

Keep yourself feeling as well as possible
There is really no need to suffer devastating withdrawal symptoms. If when you reduce the drug you feel the symptoms coming back, you could continue taking enough of it to keep yourself reasonably comfortable, and meanwhile work on your diet and general health some more before cutting down any further. It can be a very long, slow process if you are severely debilitated. I reduced my own antidepressant over two years, with the aid of a nail file.

Taking drugs? Be better informed
There are now many popular books giving a comprehensive guide to drugs and over-the-counter medicines with the side-effects clearly explained. It is wise to check yourself regularly as side-effects do not always appear until you have been taking a drug for some time. These books also discuss any circumstances under which the drug should not be taken and whether any other checks such as blood tests should be made.

Why didn't I know about the drug-free approach before?
Like so many others, I would have followed the drug-free route from the beginning if only I had known about it. I was distressed and angry that I, as a health professional, could have been so disastrously unaware. I was angry at the doctors too until I realised that they knew no more about it than I did myself.

Drugs are also the commercial approach to illness
The fact is that there are no fortunes to be made from natural medicine; it faces much opposition, especially nutritional medicine. Things are beginning to change for the better but progress is still slow. Few people fully appreciate the devastating human consequences of the present situation.

WHICH PRACTITIONER?

What does a dietitian do?
Dietitians are trained in orthodox nutrition and work with doctors to treat those conditions which are medically recognised. They also give instruction on healthy eating.

What is a nutritionist?
A nutritionist has a degree in orthodox nutrition and usually works in research or in the food industry.

What is a nutritional therapist?
Nutritional therapy is alternative nutrition, part of complementary medicine. Nutritional therapists use individually tailored diets and vitamin and mineral supplements which accelerate natural healing. This approach is highly effective in most conditions. The symptoms drop gently away without the need for drugs.

Nutritional medicine (clinical ecology)

The demand for this approach is growing fast. These doctors look at the diet and lifestyle first. They consider allergies, candida and nutritional deficiencies. They use anti-fungal drugs where necessary and most have safe and effective desensitising treatments for food intolerance, chemical sensitivities and inhaled allergens. The majority of those in the UK work privately at present; very few are actually employed by the National Health Service.

Nutritional Testing Laboratories
There are now private laboratories which support nutritional therapy and nutritional medicine. They test for deficiencies of vitamins, minerals, essential fatty acids and very much more.

Can I get help if I cannot afford private medicine?
In Britain it is now possible to be referred free of charge via the National Health Service to the private doctors and laboratories

specialising in nutritional medicine. See Useful Addresses at the end of the book.

Homoeopathy

Homoeopathic principles date back to antiquity and are based on the principle that 'like cures like'. It has been found that minute doses of a substance which, in larger doses, could cause a particular problem, can also be very effective in treating it. It functions by stimulating a healing response and can work extremely well; much depends on the skill of the homoeopath in matching the remedy to the individual. Once you are firmly established on a regenerative diet like the Hay diet, the other complementary therapies can work very much more effectively.

Naturopathy

Modern naturopaths are highly trained independent practitioners of alternative medicine who are able to examine their patients themselves and make their own diagnosis. In Britain they also issue their own Sickness or Incapacity Certificates which are recognised by the Departments of Health and Social Security. Their work focuses on improving general health without the use of drugs, mainly by detoxifying the body.

They also consider individual nutritional, emotional and environmental influences and advocate an all-round healthy lifestyle with hydrotherapy and exercise. Many naturopaths are also qualified osteopaths or accupuncturists. Naturopaths in Germany are even more highly trained and have equal status with medical practitioners. In the USA, while still undergoing long and rigorous training, they are required in most states to work under the supervision of a doctor of medicine.

SCEPTICAL?

If you have never tried natural medicine, especially nutritional treatment, you may think I am making extravagant claims for it.

However, many an honest but disbelieving doctor or scientist, setting out to disprove it, has had a change of heart to rival that of St Paul and has joined the ranks of its most ardent supporters!

**EXPERIENCE THE POWER OF
NUTRITIONAL MEDICINE**

AT MEALTIMES

Once a day
One extra strong multivitamin and mineral tablet
containing at least 25 mg vitamin B complex

Twice a day
Vitamin C one gram (1,000 mg)

Two or three times a day
Evening primrose oil one gram (2 × 500 mg capsules)

Gradually reduce the supplements when you feel better

The treatment given in the box is a short-term formula which can be highly effective in a variety of situations. You will be surprised at how fast it can work:

- If you feel an infection coming on you can often nip it in the bud.
- It can prevent a cold or 'flu, or at least shorten its life.
- It can relieve the pain of a dental abscess.
- It can hasten recovery from an injury or operation.
- It can help you over an emotional shock or any other highly stressful episode.

How does it work?

These supplements work together as a team to boost your immune defences and to support the adrenal glands during times of stress.

Evening primrose oil, despite its gentle name, is definitely anti-viral and quite formidably powerful if you take enough of it. It was known long ago as 'the King's cure-all' and its benefits are too numerous to mention.

The vitamin and mineral tablets give you strength and a much-needed lift, and they enhance the effect of evening primrose oil.

Vitamin C is also anti-viral and a natural antibiotic.

Don't forget to get the food right first

- Remember that processed food hinders recovery.
- Drink plenty of fluid, especially water.
- Glucose drinks are out.
- Keep to natural food, especially fresh fruit and salad. Fresh fruit or vegetable juices can make a tremendous difference to the way you feel. They will greatly accelerate your recovery.

IMPORTANT POINTS

1 The ordinary multivitamin and mineral tablets sold in pharmacies are not strong enough for people who are unwell, so make sure you get the high potency variety, from a health food shop. Quest 'SUPER Once A Day' tablets contain 50 mg vitamin B complex and are very widely available. A pharmacist could order them for you if necessary.

2 If you have problems taking ordinary vitamin C you could try Natural Food State Vitamin C. It is better absorbed so you need less of it.

3 If you take vitamins long term you need to be aware of the side-effects as some are stored and can build up to an overdose in the body, especially vitamins A and D. A consumer guide is suggested in Further Reading.

Keep a look-out for special offers on vitamins and evening primrose oil in the health food shops. These supplements can also be ordered from the food supplement companies listed in Useful Addresses.

Useful Addresses

Help, information and support

Action for M.E. and Chronic Fatigue
PO Box 1302, Wells, Somerset BA5 2WE.
Tel: 0891 122976 (24-hour information line, 39p per minute cheap rate, 49p at other times); (M.E. helpline); 01749 670799 (ordinary calls for general enquiries).
Information on local contacts and self-help groups; a large range of very helpful factsheets; excellent magazine, giving help from doctors and patients, the latest research and much more.

The Royal London Homoeopathic Hospital
Great Ormond Street, London W1N 3HT.
Tel: 0171 837 8833
NHS help for candida, food allergies and M.E., including in-patient beds for people outside the area. The natural approach to many other problems. GP referral required.

The Hahneman Society (also at the above address)
Send for a free leaflet, 'How to get Homoeopathic Treatment on the NHS' and for a list of homoeopathic doctors.

The Breakspear Hospital
Belswains Lane, Hemel Hempstead, Herts. HP3 9HP.
Tel: 01442 61333
Outpatients only. They have a guest house for people who live far away. Treatment for candida, allergy, food intolerance and chemical sensitivities. Over 60 per cent of their patients are funded by the NHS.

The Community Health Council
There is one in every locality (the address is in your telephone

directory). They listen sympathetically and help to sort out diffi-culties with GPs or hospitals.

Society for the Promotion of Nutritional Therapy
PO Box 47, Heathfield, East Sussex TN21 8ZX.
Tel: 01435 867007
A campaigning organisation with a regular magazine. Send SAE and £1 for a list of practitioners in your area.

Institute for Optimum Nutrition
Blades Court, Deodar Road, Putney, London SW15 2NU.
Tel: 0181 877 9993
Send £2 for a register of nutritional therapists. A lively and helpful colour magazine available by subscription. Home study courses in nutrition also available. This is a training school for nutritional therapists.

General Council and Register of Naturopaths
Goswell House, 2 Goswell Road, Street, Somerset BA16 0JG.
Tel: 01458 840072
Send SAE and £2.50 cheque/postal order for register.

National Institute of Medical Herbalists
56 Longbrook Street, Exeter, Devon EX4 6AH.
Tel: 01392 426022
Send large SAE and 29p stamp for register.

Society of Homoeopaths
2 Artisan Road, Northampton NN1 4HU.
Tel: 01604 21400
Send large SAE for information sheet and register.

Bristol Cancer Help Centre
Grove House, Cornwallis Grove, Clifton, Bristol BS8 4PG.
Tel: 0117 980 9505 (helpline); 0117 980 9500 (centre information)
The natural approach, including diet. Information on nutrition and cancer available from database.

The Hyperactive Children's Support Group
71 Whyke Lane, Chichester, West Sussex PO19 2LD.
Help for hyperactive and allergic children. Extremely helpful journal.

The Vegetarian Society UK
Parkdale, Dunham Road, Altrincham, Cheshire WA14 4QG.
You can send for their excellent information sheets.

The Bournemouth Complementary Medical Practice
Ridge Cottage, 20 Ferncroft Road, Bournemouth, Dorset BH10 6BY.
Write for a list of practitioners who use the six-hour glucose tolerance test for hypoglycaemia (available privately only).

The College of Nutritional Medicine
Eastbank, New Church Road, Smithills, Greater Manchester BL1 5QP.
Tel: 01884 255059
Courses for professional training in nutritional therapy, including correspondence courses.

UNITED STATES OF AMERICA

American Academy of Environmental Medicine
4510 W. 89th Street, Prairie Village, Kansas 66207.
Tel: (913) 341 3625

American Association of Naturopathic Physicians
PO Box 20386, Seattle, WA 98102.
Tel: (206) 323 7610

The American Dietetic Association
216 W. Jackson, Suite 800, Chicago, Ill 60606.
Tel: (312) 899 0040

Doctors specialising in allergy and nutritional medicine

A few work directly for the NHS. GP fundholders may refer people to private doctors themselves; non-fundholders may refer patients via the local Health Commission. If you are paying, you can consult a private doctor without a GP referral if necessary. Most are happy to discuss the problem on the telephone first.

British Society for Allergy and Environmental Medicine
PO Box 28, Totton, Southampton SO40 2ZA.
Ask your GP to write for a list of doctors with a special interest in nutritional medicine.

Biolab Medical Unit
The Stone House, 9 Weymouth Street, London W1N 3FF.
Tel: 0171 6365959
Private consultations in nutritional medicine. Laboratory tests for body levels of vitamins, minerals, essential fatty acids, and much more. A private laboratory. Patients can also be funded by the NHS.

Other therapies

Local Hospital Physiotherapy Departments
Aromatherapy and acupuncture are becoming more widely practised by hospital physiotherapists, especially in connection with chronic pain; but whatever your problem, it is worth enquiring of your GP or hospital.

Local Colleges of Further Education
Some now run courses in holistics, including aromatherapy, reflexology and massage. Supervised treatments given by students are at much reduced prices.

Privately run training courses in alternative therapies
These may provide similar opportunities for the above treatments, plus herbal medicine, naturopathy, osteopathy, acupuncture and homoeopathy.

Here's Health magazine
Comprehensive lists of private training courses. There may be one near where you live. It also contains details of how to find a private practitioner.

Food supplement companies

All the food supplement companies are user-friendly and will always answer any queries. You can order by telephone using a credit card. Their mail order service is fast and efficient. Goods usually arrive in 24–48 hours. Packing charges are minimal.

Cytoplan Ltd
Unit 8, Hanley Workshops, Hanley Road, Hanley Swan, Worcestershire WR8 0DX.
Tel: 01684 310099 (information line)
Natural food state vitamins and minerals including vitamin C. Food grade linseed oil (flax seed oil). Loose psyllium husks.

Higher Nature Ltd
The Nutrition Centre, Burwash Common, East Sussex TN19 7LX.
Tel: 0891 615522 (nutrition information)
Telephone line staffed by qualified nutritional therapists, weekdays 11am–7pm, 39p per minute cheap rate, 49p at other times.

Biocare
Lakeside, 180 Lifford Lane, Kings Norton, Birmingham, B30 3NT.
Tel: 0121 433 3727
Digestive enzymes: Glutenzyme and Prolactazyme.

Lamberts Healthcare Ltd
1 Lamberts Road, Tunbridge Wells, Kent TN2 3EQ.
Tel: 01892 552119
Most of Lamberts' products are available on British NHS prescription at the doctor's discretion, including digestive enzymes

and caprylic acid. Contact Lamberts to ask what is available, as the situation can change and doctors and pharmacists are usually not very familiar with these products.

Quest Vitamins Ltd
Venture Way, Aston Science Park, Birmingham B7 4AP.
Tel: 0121 3590056
Free information line staffed by qualified nutritionists.

Metabolics Ltd
5 Eastcott Common, Devizes, Wiltshire SN10 4PL.
Tel: 01380 812799
Huge range of herbal tinctures, nutritional supplements, anti-fungal preparations and products from Thorne Research USA which are specially formulated for easy tolerance. Private consultations also available.

G & G Products
175 London Road, East Grinstead, West Sussex RH19 1YY.
Tel: 01342 312811; 01342 323016 (24-hour order line)
Vitality News, a very helpful quarterly newsheet, is issued to customers.

Health check

Multimedia project centred on a free paper and involving a monthly radio programme, teletext and the internet. Organised by the *Journal of Alternative and Complementary Medicine.* Free paper available from health food shops, focusing on highly effective drug-free help for a different health problem each month—e.g. asthma, arthritis, allergies, candida.

Other free papers are usually available monthly from health food shops and they can be quite helpful.

Further Reading

Titles marked with an asterisk contain scientific references.

The Hay diet

Complete Food Combining, Peter and Donna Thompson, Bloomsbury, 1996.
The Food Combiner's Meal Planner, Kathryn Marsden, Thorsons, 1994.
Food Combining, Tim Spong and Vicki Peterson, Prism Press, 1991.
The Food Combining Cookbook, Erwina Lidolt, Thorsons, 1987.
*The Food Combining Diet, Kathryn Marsden, Thorsons, 1993.
Food Combining for Health, Doris Grant and Jean Joice, Thorsons, 1984.
The Food Combining for Health Cookbook, Jean Joice and Jackie LeTissier, Thorsons, 1994.
Food Combining for Life, Doris Grant, Thorsons, 1995.
Food Combining for Vegetarians, Jackie LeTissier, Thorsons, 1992.
The Hay Diet Menu Planner, Suzanne Gibbs, Foulsham, 1994.
A New Health Era, Dr William Howard Hay, Harrap, 1933.
The Raw Energy Food Combining Book, Leslie Kenton, Ebury Press, 1996.
The Superfoods Diet Book, Michael Van Straten and Barbara Griggs, Dorling Kindersley, 1992.

Hypoglycaemia

*Complete Nutrition, Dr Michael Sharon, Prion, 1989.
*Hypoglycaemia, Marilyn Light, Keats, 1983.

Hypoglycaemia: A Better Approach, Dr Paavo Airola, Health Plus, 1977 (available from the Nutricentre—see address on p. 158).

Hypoglycaemia: The Disease Your Doctor Won't Treat, Jeraldine Saunders and Dr Harvey M. Ross, Pinnacle Books, 1980 (available from the Nutricentre—see p. 158).

*Low Blood Sugar, Martin Budd, Thorsons, 1984.

Mental Health and Illness, Dr Carl Pfeiffer and Patrick Holford, ION Press, 1996.

Mental Illness: Not all in the mind, Patrick Holford (ed.), ION Press, 1995.

*Nutrition for Your Nerves, Dr H. Newbold, Keats, 1993.

Sugar Blues, William Dufty, Warner Books, 1975 (available from the Nutricentre—see p. 158). *About sugar itself.*

Sugar-Free Cooking, Elbie Lebrecht, Thorsons, 1994.

Sugar-Free Desserts, Drinks and Ices, Elbie Lebrecht, Faber & Faber, 1993.

Candida

Beat Candida Cookbook, Erica White, White's Food Supplement Supplies, 1991.

Boost Your Immune System, Jennifer Meek, ION Press, 1996.

Candida, Angela Kilmarton, Bloomsbury, 1995.

Candida Albicans: Could Yeast Be Your Problem?, Leon Chaitow, Thorsons, 1991.

Feeling Tired All the Time, Dr Joe Fitzgibbon, Gill & McMillan, 1993.

The Practical Guide to Candida, Jane McWhirter, All Hallows House Foundation, 1995 (distributed by Green Library, tel: 0171 385 0012).

Food allergy and intolerance

Are You Allergic? Dr William G. Crook, Professional Books, 1974.

Arthritis: The Allergy Connection, Dr John Mansfield, Thorsons, 1990.

Asthma Epidemic, Dr John Mansfield, Thorsons, 1997.

Food Allergy and Food Intolerance, Dr Jonathan Brostoff and Linda Gamlin, Bloomsbury, 1989.

The Migraine Revolution, Dr John Mansfield, Thorsons, 1986.

Not All in the Mind, Dr Richard Mackarness, Thorsons, 1976.

Toxicity

Beyond Cellulite, Nicole Ronsard, Vermilion Arrow, 1993.

Cancer and Leukaemia: An Alternative Approach, Jan De Vries, Mainstream Publishing, 1988.

Diet, Nutrition and the Prevention of Chronic Diseases, World Health Organisation Technical Report Series no. 797 Report of the WHO Study Group 1990, HMSO.

E for Additives, Maurice Hanssen, Thorsons, 1987.

Food, Teens and Behaviour, Barbara Reed, Natural Press, 1983.

Good Enough to Eat, Michael Bateman, Sinclair Stevenson, 1991.

Nutrition and Physical Degeneration, D. D. S. Price and A. Weston Price, Keats, 1990.

The Saccharine Disease, T. L. Cleave, Keats, 1974.

A Time to Heal, Beata Bishop, Penguin, 1996.

Toxaemia Explained, Dr John H. Tilden, Health Research, 1960.

Toxemia: The Basic Cause of Disease, Dr John H. Tilden, Natural Hygiene Press, PO Box 3060, Tampa, Florida 33630, USA.

Toxic Psychiatry, Peter Breggin, Fontana 1993.

Unfit for Human Consumption, Richard Lacey, Souvenir Press, 1991.

Healthy nutrition

A Doctor in the Wilderness, Dr Walter Yellowlees, Janus Publishing, 1993.

The Eskimo Diet: How to Avoid a Heart Attack, Dr Reg Saynor and Dr Frank Ryan, Ebury Press, 1990.

*Evening Primrose Oil, Judy Graham, Thorsons, 1984.

Fat Chances and Slim Hopes, Joanne Corley, TWM Publishing, 1996 (available by ringing Tel: 01734 844337).

The Fats We Need to Eat, Jeanette Ewin, Thorsons, 1995.

*Healing Foods, Dr Rosy Daniel, Thorsons, 1996.

Immune Power, Jennifer Meek, Optima, 1990.

*Let's Get Well, Adele Davis, Thorsons, 1966.

Light as a Feather, Linda Robson and Patrick Holford, Vision Video, 1994 (videotape).

The Whole Health Manual, Patrick Holford, Thorsons, 1988.

Zest for Life, Barbara Griggs, Ebury Press, 1989.

Complementary medicine

Atlas of Anatomy, Marshall Cavendish Books, 1985.

The Consumer Guide to Vitamins, Angela Dowden and Graham Lacey, Pan Books, 1996.

Food and Healing, Anne Marie Colbin, Ballantine Books, 1986.

The Food Scandal, Caroline Walker and Geoffrey Cannon, Century, 1985.

Homoeopathy: Medicine for the 21st Century, Dana Ullman, Thorsons, 1988.

Medicines, Dr I. K. M. Morton and Dr J. M. Hall, Parragon Books, 1995.

*Naturopathic Medicine, Roger Newman Turner, Thorsons, 1984.

The Optimum Nutrition Workbook, Patrick Holford, ION Press, 1988.

Principles of Nutritional Therapy, Linda Lazarides, Thorsons, 1996.

The Unmasking of Medicine, Ian Kennedy, Granada 1983.

Magazine

Here's Health. Popular and very helpful monthly magazine which supports the approach taken in this book. Available from larger newsagents, health food shops and by ordering through local newsagents. To take out a subscription, contact Here's Health Subscriptions, Tower Publishing Services, Tower House, Sovereign Park, Lathkill Street, Market Harborough, Leicestershire LE16 9EF. Tel: 01858 468888.

How to obtain the books listed above

American books not available in UK bookshops can be ordered by post from: The Nutricentre, 7 Park Crescent, London W1N 3HE. Tel: 0171 436 5122 *or* Revital, 35 High Road, Willesden, London NW10 2TE. Freefone: 0800 252 875.

Out of print books may be obtained from your local public library or will be listed on their computer. If they do not have a particular book they may be able to obtain it for you from another library. Scientific papers can also be requested from them.

Bookfinder service: Many W. H. Smith bookshops have special bookfinder computers which show you a list of books on any given subject on the screen. The list can also be printed out for you. You can order any book by telephone: 0345 581549 (Monday to Saturday, 10 a.m. to 7 p.m.) for the price of a local call. It will be sent to your local branch for collection.

Mail order: Dillons bookshops operate a mail order service from their main London shop: Dillons Mail Order Department, 82 Gower Street, London WC1E 6EQ. Tel: 0171 636 1577. Fax: 0171 580 7680 (in UK); 44 171 580 7680 (from outside UK).
email: orders@.dillons.co.uk